Topics in Nurse Prescribing

r University
ng Information Services

TANDARD LOA

Topics in Nurse Prescribing

British Journal of
Community Nursing monograph

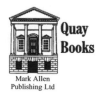

Quay
Books

Mark Allen
Publishing Ltd

Quay Books Division, Mark Allen Publishing Limited, Jesses Farm, Snow Hill, Dinton, Wiltshire, SP3 5HN

British Library Cataloguing-in-Publication Data
A catalogue record is available for this book

© Mark Allen Publishing Ltd 2002
ISBN 1 85642 224 0

Printed in the UK by Cromwell Press, Trowbridge, Wiltshire

Contents

List of contributors

Lynn Basford is Head of Nursing, School of Nursing and Community Studies, University of Derby.

Alison Bentley is District Nurse Team Leader, Elderly Hospital at Home Team, Croydon and Surrey Downs NHS Community Trust, Croydon.

Jenny Bentley is Lecturer, Florence Nightingale School of Nursing and Midwifery, King's College, London.

Dianne Bowskill is Health Lecturer, School of Nursing, Derby Royal Infirmary, Derby.

Nicky Brooks is Research Co-ordinator in Primary Care, De Montfort University, Leicester.

Willie Doherty is Clinical Nurse Specialist, Continence Service, Park Drive Health Centre, East and North Hertfordshire NHS Trust, Baldock.

Xena Dion is Clinical Effectiveness Manager, New Forest PCT, Fordingbridge Hospital, Fordingbridge, Hampshire.

Margaret Edwards is Lecturer, Florence Nightingale School of Nursing and Midwifery, King's College, London.

Jenny Gallagher is Consultant in Dental Public Health, Guy's, King's and St Thomas' Dental Institute, King's College, London and Lambeth, Southwark and Lewisham Health Authority, London.

Joanna Ibarra is Programme Coordinator, Community Hygiene Concern, London.

Elizabeth Kilty is Lead Community Practice Teacher and Board Nurse, South Leicestershire PCT.

Janice Lee is a Clinical Nurse Specialist in Stoma Care, North Tyneside Primary Care NHS Trust, Wallsend Health Centre, Wallsend, Tyne and Wear.

Christopher Maggs was formerly Professor of Nursing Practice and Development, De Montfort University, Leicester.

Christine Otway is Lead Community Practice Teacher, Eastern Leicester PCT.

Jill Peters is Dermatology Nurse Practitioner/Community Liaison Nurse, Chelsea and Westminster NHS Trust, London.

Claire Rashid is Senior Nurse Professional Development, Leicester and Rutland Healthcare Trust, The Tower's Hospital, Humberstone, Leicestershire.

Chris Rodden is Clinical Trainer, Ayrshire and Arran Primary Care Trust, Ayr, Scotland.

Jean Rowe is Nurse Adviser, Lambeth, Southwark and Lewisham Health Authority, London.

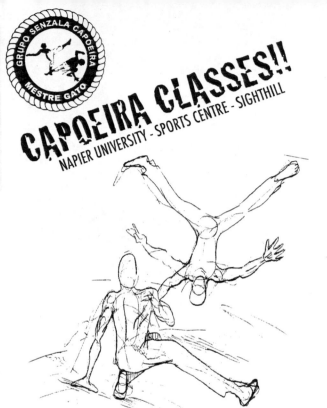

CAPOEIRA CLASSES!!

NAPIER UNIVERSITY - SPORTS CENTRE - SIGHTHILL

THURSDAYS 5.15pm - 6.15pm   FROM 24th FEBRUARY

CAPOEIRA = BRAZILIAN ART FORM = MARTIAL ART + DANCE + MUSIC + ACROBATICS = ALL IN ONE!!

VENUE:

Sports Centre Napier University Sighthill Campus

FREE CLASS ON 24th FEBRUARY

Foreword

It is sixteen years since the Cumberlege Report (Department of Health and Social Security [DHSS], 1986) first recommended prescribing by nurses as a means of improving patient care and maximising healthcare resources. Since then the Medicinal Products: Prescription by Nurses etc Act 1992 has been enacted with all district nurses and health visitors being trained as independent prescribers from 1999. More recently, the Health and Social Care Act 2001 permitted the extension of prescribing to other nurses and allied healthcare professionals including pharmacists. In the wake of this Act, the first nurse prescribers using the *Nurse Prescribers' Extended Formulary* which includes all the General Sales List (GSL) and Pharmacy only (P) medicines will enter practice during the spring of 2002. Rapid progress is also being made to establish the framework for supplementary prescribing both by nurses and pharmacists in the field of chronic disease management, with the consultation process due to be completed in the summer of 2002. It is against this background that this book is so timely, providing chapters of great relevance to prescribing district nurses and health visitors written by experts.

While a number of chapters address topics of interest to all nurse prescribers, some chapters have greater relevance to district nurses or health visitors. Xena Dion's chapter (*Chapter 5*) highlights the importance of sound record keeping not only on the grounds of professional accountability but as a means of promoting good communication across the care team. This chapter reminds practitioners that with the number of clinical negligence cases ever increasing, a high standard of record keeping will promote patient safety and also safeguard the nurse regarding their execution of professional responsibility. The advice regarding the key imperatives of good record keeping should be heeded by all practitioners. *Chapters 9, 10, 11* and *13* provide evidence of the benefits of nurse prescribing both to patients and the prescribing nurses, while also reminding readers of the challenges which need to be met as nurse prescribing continues to develop. The importance of continuing professional education together with ongoing local support in the form of clinical supervision or peer support where possible are highlighted. In contrast, Jenny Gallagher and Jean Rowe's chapter regarding the neglected area of oral health and Jill Peters' chapter regarding the management of dry skin provide key material to inform effective prescribing practice regardless of discipline.

The particular interests of district nurses are addressed in five chapters with the in depth exploration of selected product groups frequently prescribed by district nurses. Thus, *Chapters 1, 2* and *8* explore the issues regarding the selection and prescription of certain appliances (stoma bags, urinary sheaths and compression hosiery), while *Chapter 6* addresses the management of constipation in housebound older people, and *Chapter 8* the management of chronic wounds. Reflecting the more limited scope for prescribing by health visitors within the context of the current district nurse/health visitor *NPF*, there are two excellent chapters by Joanna Ibarra regarding the management of head lice and threadworms.

Invariably, a book of this type can be accused of neglecting important topics, however, the intention of this volume is to set the scene for a series of books which together will provide a comprehensive overview of topics. This first volume provides well-researched, informative chapters addressing important topics for current nurse prescribers. It should be useful both as a reference text for practising district nurses and health visitors and as a key educational text for those studying to become district nurses and health visitors.

Alison While
Professor of Community Nursing
Florence Nightingale School of Nursing and Midwifery
King's College, London
April 2002

1

Nurse prescribing in practice: patient choice in stoma care

Janice Lee

This chapter examines the choices facing nurse prescribers when selecting items for stoma management. Studies have estimated that there are up to 100,000 people with a stoma in England and Wales, and stoma care therefore forms a significant part of community nursing caseloads. The enormous range of available items means that both patient and prescriber are likely to have difficulty selecting the correct device. Patient preference, comfort and pricing all play a part in stoma appliance selection.

The long-awaited arrival of nurse prescribing for all appropriately qualified community nurses means that, among a range of other items, they are eligible to prescribe stoma appliances and associated products. However, there are some 147 pages of these products listed in Part IXC of the *Drug Tariff.* When confronted with this enormous range and combination of appliances — that seems to expand on a monthly basis — this may be confusing for the nurse prescriber. There has been a significant increase during the last decade in the number of stoma appliance manufacturing companies, which now number more than ten. Each of these companies manufactures its own unique range of stoma appliances and associated products.

As a result, patients and prescribers are provided with an excellent, if sometimes overwhelming choice of stoma appliances suited to a range of situations.

Choosing a stoma appliance can be especially difficult for patients immediately following surgery to form a stoma. Because of the nature of the surgery, the patients are required to choose a stoma appliance to wear when initially they have little or no experience of what they require. As a result they may try several different types and styles of stoma appliances before selecting one they like and feel comfortable wearing. Devlin (1985) emphasises:

The provision of a satisfactory appliance is essential to the

> *patient with a stoma, not only for physical but also for psychological reasons.*

Estimates suggest that there are up to 100,000 people who have a colostomy, ileostomy or a urostomy in England and Wales, approximately 65% of whom have a permanent stoma (Black, 1997). The greatest proportion of these patients have a colostomy, followed by an ileostomy, with the least number having an urostomy. There are smaller numbers of patients who have both a faecal and urinary stoma (Borwell, 1996; Black, 1997). Statistics suggest that the number of patients who have a colostomy, ileostomy or urostomy has fluctuated little during the past decade (Black, 1997). Although current surgical techniques are theoretically helping to reduce the number of permanent stomas being created, there has been an increase in the number of patients with a temporary stoma (National Health Service [NHS] Executive, 1997).

Stomas

Stoma is the Greek word for mouth or opening. There are three main types of stoma (*Figure 1.1*):

Colostomy: formed when the colon is raised at any position of the colon and sited on any part of abdominal wall. Colostomies may be permanent or temporary. The surgery may be carried out because of cancer of the colon, diverticular disease, Crohn's disease, irradiation damage, obstruction, ischaemic bowel, trauma or congenital conditions.

Ileostomy: formed from the ileum (usually the terminal ileum) and positioned in the right iliac area. Ileostomies may also be permanent or temporary. Surgery may be carried out because of inflammatory bowel disease (eg. Crohn's disease and ulcerative colitis), familial adenomatous polyposis, carcinoma, irradiation damage, obstruction, trauma or necrotising enterocolitis.

Urostomy: these stomas are usually permanent. They involve diversion of the urinary tract and are generally positioned in the right iliac area. Surgery may be carried out because of cancer of the bladder or urethra, spinal column disorders ('neurogenic bladder'), or urinary incontinence.

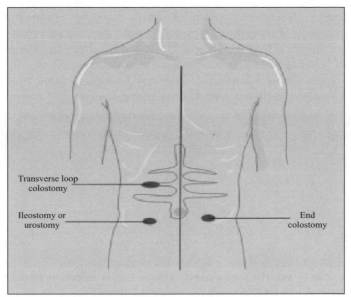

Transverse loop
colostomy

Ileostomy or
urostomy

End
colostomy

Figure 1.1: Location of different types of stoma

Stoma appliances

There are two basic categories of stoma appliances, both of which are available with clear or opaque coverings. Both categories have a flange that is designed to protect the skin surrounding the stoma, as well as allowing the stoma to be enclosed within the pouch. The pouch collects the urine or faeces, depending on the type of stoma. One-piece appliances (*Figures 1.2, 1.3* and *1.5*) consist of a flange and pouch manufactured together. Two–piece appliances (*Figure 1.4*) consist of a flange — which is cut to fit and adheres round the stoma site and requires changing every 3–5 days — with an outer pouch which is secured by clipping to the flange. The advantage of a two-piece system is that the outer pouch can be changed frequently as required, while minimising the discomfort of repeated flange changes.

Closed appliances are used for collecting formed stool and are mainly (although not exclusively) used for patients who have a colostomy. The appliance must be changed when approximately half-full; up to three times per day depending on stool consistency and output. A drainable appliance is used in the immediate post-operative period for patients with a colostomy and is usually used postoperatively and continually thereafter for patients with an ileostomy. Drainable appliances must also be emptied when approximately half-full. The pouch should be changed every 3–4 days, or sooner if leakage occurs. Urostomy pouches are designed to collect urine and have an outlet tap at the bottom to allow emptying when approximately half-full. This may be five or more times per day. Urostomy appliances should be changed every 3–5 days.

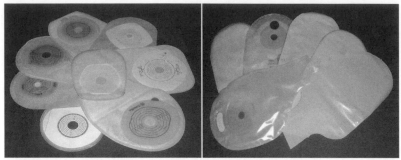

Figure 1.2: A selection of closed one-piece stoma pouches

Figure 1.3: A selection of drainable stoma pouches

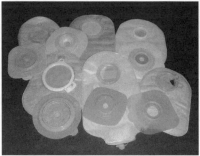

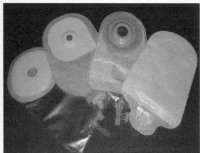

Figure 1.4: A selection of two-piece stoma pouches

Figure 1.5: A selection of one-piece urostomy pouches

Complications

A frequent problem common to all types of stoma is skin irritation. This may occur as a result of faeces or urine leaking onto the peristomal area, either because the stoma has altered in shape or size, or because the appliance flange has not been cut to correspond with the alteration. Skin irritation may also occur because of a reaction to the materials in the flange or pouch material, or an associated item used on the peristomal skin, such as deodoriser or protective powder.

Cost considerations

Stoma care appliances and associated products are in the top twenty of the most frequently prescribed items, accounting for 1.3 million prescriptions dispensed in England in 1999. The approximate cost of these was £96 million (Kendall, 2000). It is essential, in order to optimise the use of the NHS budget, that careful consideration is given to the cost of stoma appliances and any associated products a patient may require before issuing a prescription.

The cost of a single one-piece standard closed appliance for a patient with a colostomy ranges from £2.00–£2.30 on the *Drug Tariff*, and the frequency of appliance change for a colostomist can range from one to four appliances per day.

The cost of a one-piece standard size drainable appliance suitable for a patient with an ileostomy ranges from £1.90–£2.50, and the frequency of appliance change for an ileostomist is every two to four days. The cost of a one-piece standard size urostomy appliance suitable for a patient with a urostomy ranges from £3.95–£4.64 per appliance. The frequency of appliance change for the urostomist is every three to four days. The cost of a flange for two-piece systems ranges from £2.29–£2.87 each, plus the cost of individual pouches which ranges from £1.05–£1.21 for a closed pouch, £1.08–£1.10 for the drainable pouch and £2.33–£2.37 for a urostomy pouch. All pouches are packaged in boxes of ten, twenty, thirty or fifty and flanges are packaged in boxes of either five or ten.

Assessment

Before the nurse prescriber issues any prescription, he/she must conduct a full assessment of the patient's condition, in order to ascertain the rationale for requiring a prescription from a nurse prescriber rather than through the usual route. During the assessment the nurse prescriber must enquire what type of stoma the patient has, and the reason why the patient requires a prescription for stoma products or associated products. It may be that the patient has run out of supplies, although experience suggests that this would be highly unusual. It is more likely that the patient may have had an increased frequency of appliance changes because of leakage, resulting in skin irritation.

It is essential that the patient identifies what type of stoma they have in order to prevent prescription of an inappropriate stoma appliance. Unlike the prescribing of many other items in the *Nurse Prescribers' Formulary* (*NPF*) (1999), it is also important for the nurse prescriber to include the patient in the choice of a suitable stoma appliance; the patient must feel comfortable and confident while wearing the appliance, and not feel restricted when carrying out his/her activities of daily living. While carrying out the patient assessment the nurse prescriber will probably take into account the cost of individual manufacturers' products before prescribing the item. If an identical product is available at a cheaper cost and is suitable for that particular wound, then the nurse prescriber may choose the cheaper of the two. However, a patient who has a stoma also has the right to choose a stoma appliance which is comfortable and suitable for his/her lifestyle and needs (Campaign for Impartial Stoma Care, 1992).

A full assessment of the stoma should include some or all of the following questions:

- Has the patient recently had surgery resulting in the formation of a stoma? If yes, what type of stoma was formed?
- What type of appliance has the patient been using?
- Has the appliance started to leak and if so is there a reason why this has occurred, eg. parastomal hernia, stenosis?
- Is there any sore skin surrounding the stoma? If yes, is it due to the stoma reducing in size or due to possible sensitivity to the patient's existing stoma appliance?
- Is the stoma situated in a skin fold or dip?
- Has the stoma prolapsed?
- Should the stoma care nurse assess the patient further before prescribing and/or following renewal of the prescription?
- If the patient has no stoma appliances left, what is the reason for this?

Making a choice

Patients who receive a prescription from a nurse prescriber will take for granted the safety and appropriateness of the products prescribed.

Since the nurse will use many sources of information when considering which products to prescribe, it is important that he/she is not unduly influenced by any particular source, but makes an objective judgement based on his/her assessment of the patient and the wound, his/her knowledge of the products and cost considerations. This onus on prescribing appropriately, free from influence or bias, is backed up by the United Kingdom Central Council for Nursing, Midwifery and Health Visiting (UKCC)'s *Code of Conduct and Standards for the Administration of Medicines* (2000). Guidance relating to influence and bias is also contained in the standards of business conduct for NHS staff, which applies to all individuals working in the NHS (Parker, 2000).

If, as a nurse prescriber, the nurse has any doubt about the suitability and type of stoma appliance or associated accessory that is being considered for prescribing, then clearly the item must not be prescribed. Assistance should be requested with the patient assessment either from the patient's general practitioner (GP) or from the local stoma care nurse who will probably know the patient well.

Conclusion

Nurse prescribing offers an opportunity for community nurses to become more actively involved than ever in patient care. It also presents a challenge to nurses who will not always be familiar with the products and procedures that they are now equipped to offer. Considering the vast range of stoma appliances and associated products listed in Part IXC of the *Drug Tariff*, it may be prudent for the nurse prescriber to enlist the assistance of the local stoma care nurse as well as the patient to guide him/her through the enormous range and combination of appliances.

Key Points

✻ Stoma appliances and associated products are among the most frequently prescribed items in the UK, accounting for 1.3 million prescriptions dispensed in England alone in 1999.

✻ A patient who has a stoma has the right to choose a stoma appliance which is comfortable and suitable for his/her lifestyle and needs.

✻ Choice of stoma appliance will also be based on the type of stoma, faecal consistency, construction material and cost.

References

Black PK (1997) Practical stoma care: a community approach. *Br J Community Health Nurs* **2**(5): 249–53

Borwell B (1996) *Managing Stoma Problems*. Professional Nurse Update

Campaign for Impartial Stoma Care (1992) *Ostomy Patients' Charter*. Campaign for Impartial Stoma Care, London

Devlin HB (1985) Living with a stoma: In Devlin HB, ed. *Stoma Care Today*. Medical Education Services, Oxford: 34–7

Kendall H (2000) What happens to a prescription? *Charter* **7**: 8–9

National Health Service Executive (1997) *Guidance on Commissioning Cancer Services. Improving Outcomes in Colorectal Cancer: The Manual*. DoH, London

National Health Service Executive (1998) *Nurse Prescribing. A Guide for Implementation*. DoH, London

Nurse Prescribers' Formulary (1999) British Medical Association and Royal Pharmaceutical Society of Great Britain, London

Parker C (2000) Nurse prescribing: basic and continuing education. *J Community Nurs* **14**(9): 10–14

United Kingdom Central Council for Nursing, Midwifery and Health Visiting (2000) *Code of Conduct and Standards for the Administration of Medicines*. UKCC, London

2

Urinary sheaths: assessment, prescription and evaluation

Willie Doherty

Urinary sheaths are a common solution to male urinary incontinence, but can be a source of much anxiety and discomfort if incorrectly fitted. This chapter discusses the process of assessment that must precede the prescription of a urinary sheath system. Assessment of bladder function and correct fitting and sizing are essential. The chapter also discusses the range of urinary sheath systems available, some of the problems that may arise in their use, and the processes of evaluation that should accompany use.

Incontinence is a common problem in the community, particularly among older people. For example, approximately 37% of patients in nursing homes are incontinent of both urine and faeces (Castleden, 1999). Among the appliances available to help male patients manage their incontinence are incontinence sheaths.

Little has been written on the use of urinary sheaths and their effectiveness in the patient with urinary incontinence despite continuing research into, and development of, new materials and designs. From the author's experience, urinary sheaths were often provided in an ad hoc way in the past. Whatever was available at the time, or whichever product had become standard for each group of nurses, was generally the sheath of choice. Patients were given sheaths to try and if they proved successful (ie. stayed in position for several hours or longer, draining urine satisfactorily and did not cause any skin irritation) they were recognised as appropriate for that patient. A prescription was than requested from the general practitioner (GP). This involved a time delay from the request of the prescription to when it was available for the patient to collect. If a urinary drainage sheath was unsuccessful, it was considered to be inappropriate for use and patients were usually given disposable pads as a means of managing their incontinence. Nevertheless, urinary sheaths accounted for 164,000 prescribed items in 1999, at a cost to the NHS of over £9 million (Department of Health, 2000).

This chapter briefly reviews the assessment processes that must precede the prescription of a sheath system, the types of sheaths available, the problems that may arise in the use of incontinence sheaths, and the proper evaluation of a sheath's effectiveness.

Nurse prescribing and continence

Nurse prescribing offers a number of benefits to the nurse and to the patient:

- improved use of both patients' and nurses' time
- improved patient care
- improved communication between team members as a result of clarification of professional responsibilities (Department of Health and Social Security [DHSS], 1989).

In the management of urinary sheath drainage systems there is the opportunity for nurses not only to try out appliances but also — on finding a suitable product — to enable patients to assume responsibility for their own care and initiate further supplies of equipment themselves. This saves patient time and leads to less nurse intervention .

Pre-assessment for fitting of urinary drainage sheath

Before assessment of a patient's suitability for a particular urine drainage system, nurses must be aware of patients' bladder functions and should perform some simple pre-assessment tasks. These include completing a frequency volume chart recording intake and output, as well as the types of fluids taken. This enables evaluation of bladder function and will help the formulation of a care plan.

A bladder scan may be appropriate to identify any residual urine that may be left in the bladder after voiding, which may require an alternative form of treatment, such as intermittent self-catheterisation. Many urology wards and clinical nurse specialists in continence care have portable bladder scanners which nurses may be able to make use of. It is also prudent for nurses to assess their patients' bowel function, as constipation may be a contributory factor in urinary incontinence.

Assessment process

All too often in the past urinary drainage sheaths have been dismissed as having failed their user and carer simply because they have been poorly fitted or incorrectly measured (Doherty, 1998). Nurses need to be aware that there are many different sizes and

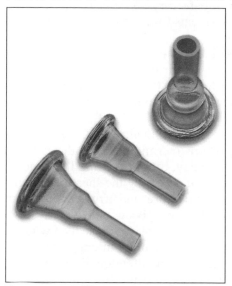

lengths of sheath available (*Figure 2.1*) to suit the majority of men, even those with penile retraction problems. Most manufacturers have produced sheath sizes in increments of 4/5mm and more recently, Manfred Sauer Gmbh have developed eleven sheath sizes, ranging from 18mm paediatric size to 40mm, in increments of 2mm (the Comfort Plus Latex Free sheath). This availability of more sheath sizes provides access to a wider range of products ensuring the optimum fit and hence reliability. The assessment process of a satisfactory urinary drainage

Figure 2.1: Different sizes of sheaths. Photograph courtesy of SIMS Portex

system for patients is initially quite time-consuming. Yet the benefits derived from correct assessment and an effective drainage system are immeasurable. As well as the physical benefits, nurses must consider the psychological advantages such as patient dignity, independence and self-esteem, which are equally important.

Patients who may be suitable for these systems need to be chosen carefully. Applying a urinary drainage sheath and attaching its associated leg bag is not an easy process. Therefore patients must ideally have either a considerable amount of finger-thumb dexterity, or a carer who will become involved in the fitting procedure. Sheath systems also demand vigilance on the part of the nurse — to ensure the products that have been supplied perform in the manner they were intended and that they do not harm the patient in any way, eg. there is no deterioration in skin condition — and motivation from patients to accept this system as a positive means of dealing with

Willie Doherty

their urinary problems. There will be occasions when the system fails, causing patients to be incontinent, but this should not influence the longer-term goal of managing the incontinence problem.

In addition to the problems that may occur as a result of the dexterity needed to fit the sheath successfully, there may also be problems relating to the very nature of the task itself. The process of assessment and fitting of a satisfactory system is an intimate procedure and some nurses and patients find this difficult (Bath *et al*, 1999) due to embarrassment.

A study conducted in 1981 found that approximately 15% of those men with spinal injury using urinary sheath systems had significant side-effects or complications (Golji, 1981). Side-effects range from reactions to the materials used to increased susceptibility to urinary tract infections (Ouslander *et al*, 1987). Patients with spinal injuries may have other methods of dealing with their bladder function problems. Some will perform intermittent self-catheterisation at regular intervals throughout the day, often requiring the removal of the urinary sheath. This process of renewing the sheath each time can cause the penile skin to become sore and irritated. A recent development in sheath manufacture has been one which has a removable tip, allowing access to the urethra, for those men who are managing their bladder function using intermittent self-catheterisation (Doherty, 1999). If strict attention is not paid to hygiene, there may be bacteria around the meatus which may be carried up the urethra to the bladder during catheterisation.

Sheath systems

There are many sheath-type systems available on prescription or for patients to purchase, and it is important that assessing nurses are aware of these. The majority of companies will send samples of their products, free of charge, with sizing guides, to any nurses who request this information. This allows nurses to try a variety of sheaths and sizes, so that patients and their carers, as well as nurses, can make informed choices on the type of appliance most suitable. Some companies provide prescription services which patients can access for delivery of their supplies. These are extremely useful for housebound patients, those without easy access to a local pharmacy or those who like the convenience of having products delivered to their homes.

It should be remembered however, that relying on the products or systems manufactured by one company may not achieve the results required for patient comfort and dignity (Bath *et al*, 1999). In 1990, Watson and Kuhn suggested that a combination of products (such as sheaths and leg bags) produced the best results with regard to successful performance.

The two-piece urinary sheath

This type of sheath (*Figure 2.2*) was developed in the early 1980s and is very successful, providing comfortable, secure urine drainage. A strip of adhesive is applied to the penis, sometimes in a spiral action and the sheath is then rolled over this adhesive area and is pressed into place. For extra security some wearers use a further anchoring device on the outside of the applied sheath, but these should only be used with extreme caution in those with spinal injuries or neurological deficit; with reduced or absent sensation, these men may not be able to feel if the device is too tight and restricting blood flow to the penis.

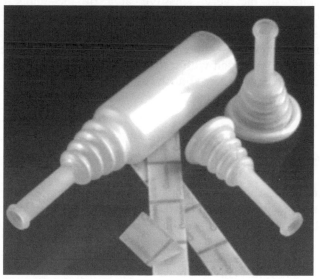

Figure 2.2: Examples of two-piece sheaths and adhesive strips. Photograph courtesy of Coloplast Ltd

Two-piece sheaths can be used in conjunction with the majority of the various urine drainage bags that are available. This type of sheath can be easily removed with soap and water and disposed of. The penis must then be washed and dried very carefully before application of a replacement. Patients and carers should be aware that any surface moisture will inactivate the adhesive of the replacement sheath. Sheaths should not be pulled to be removed, but gently rolled away from the base of the penis. Neither should they be cut off with scissors, as this is a dangerous practice.

The one-piece urinary sheath

Although there are various sheaths available which require an application of an adhesive prior to fitting, there have been many improvements to the quality of adhesive over the last few years, and several one-piece sheaths with an inner coating of adhesive have been developed (Medical Devices Agency [MDA], 2000) (*Figure 2.3*). The adhesive layer comes into contact with the skin of the penis as the sheath is rolled into place. Most one-piece sheaths do not have adhesive on the initial, unrolled part of the sheath, so as to avoid sticking to the very sensitive area of the glans penis. This non-adhesive area can expand, so may be useful in coping with a flush of urine in those who expel urine quickly, or those patients who void by external compression of their bladder. Some one-piece sheaths are provided with a disposable applicator and some have a thicker layer of material at the outlet end to avoid the problem of kinking, which can cause leakage.

Problems with sheath drainage systems

The major problem with sheath drainage systems appears to be that of the sheath falling off (Bath *et al*, 1999). However, there are other issues which nurses must take into consideration. Together with those outlined below, there is the possibility of increased susceptibility to urinary tract infections, due to the colonisation of the urinary tract (Jayachandran *et al*, 1985).

One- and two-piece sheaths are manufactured in a range of materials including latex and silicone. Some patients may have allergy problems with either of these materials. It may be advisable to perform a simple patch test on a sensitive area of the skin, such as the forearm, to assess any potential allergic reaction. Patients must be made aware of allergies or skin reactions, and given instructions as to what to do if this happens, ie. removing the sheath immediately and contacting their relevant district nurse or immediate colleague. There are three distinct types of reaction that may occur on the application or continual use of sheaths: irritation, immediate hyper-sensitivity and delayed hypersensitivity.

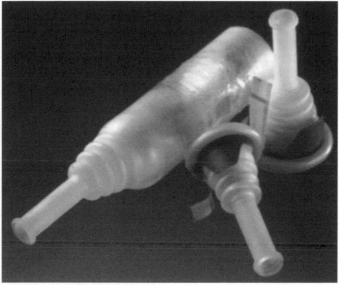

Figure 2.3: Examples of one-piece urinary sheaths. Photograph courtesy of Coloplast Ltd

Irritation

Bath *et al* (1999) have stated that irritation is a non-allergic reaction that tends to happen almost immediately after the sheath has been applied or up to several hours later. It is recognised as pink or red discolouration of the skin where the sheath or adhesive were applied. Nurses must inform carers and patients, who may not have worn or used this type of product before, that this may be a possibility and that should it occur, the appliance should be removed immediately and the area washed gently and dried thoroughly to remove any residual adhesive. This type of sheath should not be applied again and the incident should be reported to the named nurse and his/her colleagues. Such a reaction should of course be recorded in the patient's notes, so that other carers do not make the mistake of using this type of product for this particular patient.

Immediate hypersensitivity

Recognised by the MDA (1996), this reaction is usually a response to a naturally-occurring protein in rubber latex and will occur approximately five to thirty minutes after the patient is exposed to the latex of the sheath. The reaction is more pronounced than irritation, and the skin appears more reddened or inflamed. The skin may also take on a smooth stretched appearance. The reaction subsides quickly when the appliance is removed. There may be some localised residual skin irritation and oedema, which can take three to twenty-four hours to resolve, depending on the health of the patient.

Delayed hypersensitivity

Delayed hypersensitivity has been recognised as a problem for some patients by Bath *et al* (1999). This is also known as contact dermatitis and can occur up to forty-eight hours after the initial application of the sheath. It generally results in the formation of blisters or papules and usually subsides after several days but can cause considerable discomfort to the patient. Nurses and carers should be made aware of the possibility of this happening and instruct patients and carers on treatment. The sheath should be removed, which may necessitate soaking in water. The affected area should be washed to remove any residue, and the area dried and left open to the air unless blisters have formed and have exuded fluid. A clean dressing draped over the affected area helps maintain patients' dignity while also permitting free circulation of air.

Although such reactions are not common, the nurse must be aware that oedema of the penis can cause problems with bladder drainage as a result of pressure on the urethra. In the event of a hypersensitive reaction, it is also important that the appropriate nurses are notified.

Fitting a urinary sheath

Once a suitable product has been agreed upon by the patient, carer and nurse, assessment of the correct size is essential. A sheath that is too small will cause soreness of the penis and possibly ulceration; one that is too large will cause ridges to form along the shaft and will eventually lead to leakage. Penile tumesence varies throughout the day and night and it is important that this is taken into consideration when measuring for the correct size.

Allowing patients to measure themselves empowers them in the decision-making process, and can save embarrassment to them and their nurses or carers. If this is not possible, the measuring or fitting of the sheath is best performed by someone known to the patient with whom he feels comfortable (Bath *et al*, 1999). Penile circumference is measured as well as length; some manufacturers provide a shorter sheath for men with retracted penises. Many companies provide measuring devices for this purpose and it is essential that the correct device is used for the accompanying product. There are several points to remember when selecting and fitting a urinary sheath (*Table 2.1*).

Table 2.1: Points to remember when selecting and fitting a urinary sheath
It is important to:
⌘ Measure correctly the length of the penis and its circumference at its widest point
⌘ Test the product for sensitivity, bearing in mind the fact that some patients are allergic to latex
⌘ Select a sheath that is easy to apply, as ease of application promotes confidence in users
⌘ Ensure the urine bag is of the correct size and that it is well supported to avoid dragging on the sheath
⌘ Adjust seating for wheelchair users, if necessary, to allow better drainage
⌘ Monitor skin condition for soreness or ulceration
⌘ Shorten pubic hair to prevent it being caught in the sheath. Do not shave the area if possible, as subsequent regrowth can cause irritation
⌘ Avoid kinking or twisting of the sheath or the drainage bag as this allows urine to pool, thereby weakening the adhesive or blocking drainage completely
⌘ Ensure products are easily available and on the *Drug Tariff*

The wheelchair user

It is essential that the wheelchair user is not only confident with the chosen sheath system used in the collection of their urine, but that any carer involved in their nursing care, is skilled in the effective application and adjustment of the sheath. This is particularly important when patients are dressed while lying on their beds prior to being transferred to their wheelchair.

It is important that there is sufficient space beneath the patient's clothing to allow drainage of urine from the sheath into its accompanying leg bag, and that this bag attachment does not cause traction on the sheath, thus causing it to come adrift. Clothing, such as trousers and underpants, must be loose enough to prevent kinking or twisting of the sheath or leg bag. Loose exercise pants or 'jogging bottoms' are ideal for this purpose, giving not only space but allowing for easy adjustment either of the leg bag via the elasticated ankle cuff, or via the waistband. Many patients have their clothing altered, with the addition of velcro or zip fasteners just below the knee allowing easy access for emptying the urine bag, or for the carer to adjust the bag fixation system. A time for extra vigilance once the sheath system has been applied, is when the patient is removed from the bed, in a hoist to the wheelchair, or from wheelchair onto a toilet or into a car. It is essential once the patient has been moved and is comfortable, that their clothing is adjusted and the drainage system monitored to ensure that the device has not slipped, come adrift from the collecting bag, and is not being pulled by the leg bag.

Urine drainage leg bags are available in various sizes from 350mls to 750mls and Manfred Sauer have manufactured a 1300ml Bendi bag which follows the contour of the lower thigh and calf. This extra capacity affords the wheelchair user considerable independence and peace of mind while away from the home situation, as they do not have to search for what may turn out to be inadequate toilet facilities when travelling. These bags can be heavy when full of urine, and require adequate support to facilitate the extra weight, otherwise the traction on the sheath may displace it.

To ensure effective drainage from the sheath into the urine bag device, the bag must be positioned securely but not tightly onto the patient's leg, a good position being the inside of the calf, or whichever area that allows the patient to empty the device independently, and remains comfortable throughout the day. Some bag securing straps have a tendency to slip and it may be advisable to try other supporting systems, such as the Bard Urisleeve leg bag holder or the Seton Continence Care Aquasleeve (see *Drug Tariff* for further information). This type of device is a double sleeve of an elasticated mesh material applied to the calf or thigh and the bag inserted into the outer part of the sleeve. These allow for the urine to be dispersed across the bag and are more discrete.

When the bag has been secured to the patient's leg it is prudent to check the position of the sheath, ie. has it come adrift in the transfer to the wheelchair? Is the sheath pointing down towards the bag ensuring effective drainage and preventing pooling of urine around the meatus? This pooling of urine can inactivate the adhesive and cause the system to fail, leading to leakage and incontinence.

There are other sheath securing devices such as foam and velcro type strips, or various types which can be applied over the sheath at the base of the penis for added security, such as the Rusch Dryaid strip, Urifix tape or the Posey sheath holder (see *Drug Tariff*). These should be used with considerable caution and not by those with reduced or altered sensation in the genital area, as they can lead to soreness and trauma. If one-piece sheaths are applied correctly after effective assessment and measurement, then extra screening devices are not required.

Evaluation

The effectiveness of a sheath and accompanying drainage bag system requires regular evaluation to ensure the proper functioning of the system and correct practice on the part of the patient and carers. Points to attend include:

❖ Is the sheath of the correct length and of a suitable material so that it does not cause irritation or tissue damage?

❖ Is the appliance being positioned correctly by the patient or carer?

❖ Does it act in an appropriate manner, collecting urine, taking it away from the penile area and storing it effectively in the prescribed leg or night drainage bag?

❖ Is the sheath or bag liable to twist, or is it unsupported by the bag straps?

Any problems during the procedure can be addressed before they lead to the failure of the system and unnecessary distress for the patient.

Conclusion

Incontinence is an embarrassing problem and many nurses appear to choose disposable incontinence pads as the first line of management. These can offer immediate solutions to management of the problem by soaking up the urine, but it still means that patients may have to sit on damp pads for several hours, depending on the level of their supported care. Urinary sheaths and their many types and sizes of drainage bags give patients back their dignity. The urine is contained, and can be disposed of relatively easily, giving patients more independence and empowering self-care. For more mobile patients, the urine drainage systems are discrete and can be concealed easily beneath trousers. This allows for more flexibility of social interaction, preventing patients from becoming isolated.

There are many issues to consider when assessing, planning, implementing and evaluating patient care. It is essential that when prescribing sheath drainage systems and their accompanying day and night drainage bags, nurses have the knowledge to support their decisions for choosing these as suitable means of managing the male patient's incontinence or bladder problems.

Key Points

* Incontinence is a common problem in both nursing homes and the community setting.

* One- or two-piece urinary sheaths are available.

* Patients can feel empowered if they are allowed to measure themselves and are able to fit their own sheaths.

* Nurses, patients and carers need to be aware of problems that can occur with sheath drainage systems, eg. irritation, hyper-sensitivity, allergic reaction.

* Finding the most appropriate sheath for individual patients has psychological as well as physical benefits.

References

Aquasleeve Seton Continence Care: A division of Seton Healthcare Group PLC, Tubiton House, Madlock Street, Oldham OL1 3HS

Bard Urisleeve leg bag holder, Bard Ltd, Forest House, Brighton Road, Crawley, West Sussex RH11 9BP

Bath J, Fader M, Patterson L (1999) Urinary sheaths and bags: making an informed choice. *Primary Health Care* **9**(7): 17–23

Burns S (2002) Size does matter — for urinary sheaths. *Urology News* **6**(3): 38

Castleden M (1999) Incontinence: diagnosis in nursing homes. *Geriatr Med* Feb: 49–50

Department of Health (2000) *Prescription Cost Analysis England 1999.* DoH, London

Department of Health and Social Security (1989) *Report of the Advisory Group on Nurse Prescribing* (Crown report). DHSS, London

Doherty W (1998) The clear advantage urinary incontinence sheath for men. *Br J Nurs* **3**(8): 393–7

Doherty W (1999) Indications for and principles of intermittent self-catheterisation. *Br J Nurs* **8**(2): 73–84

Golji H (1981) Complications of external condom drainage. *Paraplegia* **19**: 189–97

Jayachandran S *et al* (1985) Complications from external (condom) urinary drainage devices. *Urology* **25**(1): 31–4

Medical Devices Agency (1996) *Latex sensitization in the health care setting (use of latex gloves).* MDA BD 9601. MDA, London

Medical Devices Agency (2000) *Self-adhesive sheaths for men using sheath systems: an evaluation.* IN6. MDA, London

Ouslander JG, Greengold B, Chen S (1987) External catheter use and urinary tract infections among incontinent male nursing home patients. *J Am Geriatr Soc* **35**: 1063–70

Sakett DL, Richardson WS, Rosenberg W, Haune RB (1997) *Evidence Based Medicine: How to practice and teach EBP.* Churchill Livingstone, Edinburgh

Watson R, Kuhn M (1990) The influence of component parts on the performance of urinary sheath systems. *J Adv Nurs* **15**(4): 417–22

3

Head lice: changing the costly chemotherapy culture

Joanna Ibarra

The revulsion prompted by the discovery of head lice on a child's head, and the money spent by the NHS each year on supplying licensed medicines for head lice, are disproportionate to the medical impact that lice have on their hosts. This chapter discusses the evidence available on the effectiveness of the commonest parasiticidal preparations, and argues the case for a more rational, simpler and cost-effective response to this common problem.

A disproportionate amount of health resources is devoted to the head louse problem in the UK, although it is of little clinical importance. The nurses, who may now obtain prescribing status for head infestation (*pediculosis capitis*) and, consequently, have a greater say in primary care expenditure on drug treatment, are in a position to argue for improved management in the twenty-first century.

Historical background

The Fisher Education Act of 1918 established a duty to provide treatment to children found to have 'defects' during inspections made at school by doctors or nurses. The presence of scabies and lice were classed as defects, now termed 'adverse medical conditions'. With the establishment of the National Health Service (NHS), a parent could obtain a prescription for a child from a general practitioner (GP) to be dispensed at no charge by a retail pharmacist. However, free treatments for use at home continued to be supplied by a registered or enrolled nurse directly to the patient's parent. The nurse often dispensed enough medication for the whole family. This facility of nurses to dispense medicines was held in relation to treatments for infestation of the person, by custom, not in law; it contravened the spirit of the 1968 Medicines Act, when introduced.

The Act is the foundation of modern regulation of the licensing and administration of medicines. All head lice treatment formulas on the market in 1968 and thereafter were obliged to seek a licence under the Act. Licensed formulas became 'P' products (restricted to pharmacy-only sale). P products can be sold over the counter (OTC) to the general public, as long as a pharmacist is available to advise, or dispensed by a pharmacist to fill a GP prescription. It shows to what extent the problem of lice was considered exceptional, because the introduction of these regulations under the Act made no difference to the nurses' traditional dispensing practices.

Health authorities (HAs) withdrew routine head inspections in the 1980s in order to cut costs (Owen, 1982) and distribution by nurses of free medication in school also ceased, requiring families to visit their GPs for treatment prescriptions. Some GPs found this unacceptably time-consuming. Indeed, in 1995 a survey of 107 GP receptionists attending training courses revealed that 57% were undertaking preparation of a prescription for head lice for the GP to sign without seeing the patient, while another 22% were handing out free head louse medication from the surgery (Hall *et al*, 1995).

From 1999, training has enabled community nurses with district nurse (DN) or health visitor (HV) qualifications to prescribe for certain medical conditions, including parasiticidals for scabies and head lice. Further service development aiming to give nurses power commensurate with their responsibilities (Department of Health [DoH], 2000a), will allow nurses with other qualifications, eg. practice nurses, to apply for prescribing rights. As with DNs and HVs before, this may merely add a legal seal to the way practice nurses already manage head lice cases. When school nurses may prescribe head louse medication, history will have come full circle.

Size of the head louse problem

Although all social classes are vulnerable irrespective of income and standards of personal hygiene, the stigma of lice persists. It leads people to seek treatment as soon as they are aware of lice in the family. The UK market in conventional pesticide medicines was worth £14.4 million in 1994/5 (Chemist & Druggist, 1995) rising to £29.7 million in 1997/8 (Purcell, 1998). Half the latter sum was spent by the NHS on approximately six million doses. Another four million doses were bought at a higher price per product in pharmacies by the general public. The total of ten million doses is the best indication there is of the number of cases. In addition, an unknown number of unlicensed chemotherapies of 'natural' origin and mechanical methods of clearing lice are in use.

Ascertaining diagnosis

All experts agree no medication should be used unless a live louse has been detected (*Table 3.1*). Active infestation is not proven by the presence of egg-like structures in the hair. Genuine louse eggs can remain fresh in appearance after successful chemotherapy, and will still 'pop' when pressed between the finger nails, even though their development has been arrested. Also secretions from the hair follicle wrapped round the hair shaft (hair muffs), a common and harmless condition, can mimic eggs.

Table 3.1: How head lice spread

Head lice are common among children and easily spread to the rest of the family and carers.

Head lice hold onto hairs with claws at the end of their six legs. Their eggs (nits) are firmly glued to hairs. Strictly speaking nits are the empty eggshells left stuck to the hair after the lice have hatched.

Anyone with hair on the scalp can catch head lice. Clean hair is no protection. Full grown lice climb rapidly through dry hair moving from person to person during close head to head contact; they cannot hop, fly or swim. Healthy lice live close to the scalp which they bite to draw blood, their sole food.

The tear-shaped egg is pin-head size and takes seven to ten days to hatch. Lice moult three times to grow, remaining on the head where they hatch until the third moult is complete, a minimum six days. Full grown lice are ready to move on as soon as the opportunity arises. This prevents inbreeding which would weaken the species.

On the other hand, many infestations are light, with ten or fewer lice on the head (Mellanby, 1942). The onset of itching is often delayed, so no-one realises the problem is there before it has spread. Research comparing the Bug Busting wet combing method (*Figure 3.1*) with visual inspection as performed traditionally by school nurses has shown that the latter produces unacceptably high numbers of false positives and negatives (De Maeseneer *et al*, 2000; Ibarra *et al*, 2000).

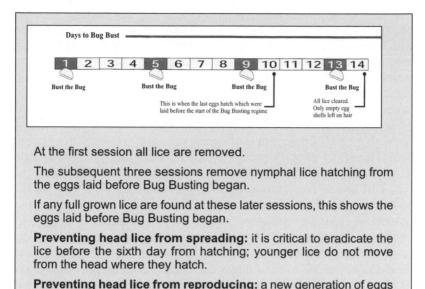

At the first session all lice are removed.

The subsequent three sessions remove nymphal lice hatching from the eggs laid before Bug Busting began.

If any full grown lice are found at these later sessions, this shows the eggs laid before Bug Busting began.

Preventing head lice from spreading: it is critical to eradicate the lice before the sixth day from hatching; younger lice do not move from the head where they hatch.

Preventing head lice from reproducing: a new generation of eggs can be laid from day seven after hatching.

Figure 3.1: Bug busting to break the life cycle

Dry or damp lice move quickly away from disturbance, evading detection. Combing wet, conditioned hair with a fine-tooth plastic comb is recommended by the DoH (2000b) as a reliable detection method because thoroughly wet lice stay still (Hase, 1931). Parents need to know about accurate detection and are encouraged to learn the skill, which, used systematically, can also clear lice. Nurses can direct parents to the Bug Buster help line and/or website run by the health charity, Community Hygiene Concern (CHC), for information.

Legal status of products

A DoH body, the Medicines Control Agency (MCA), regulates the efficacy, safety and quality of medicinal products, which are defined as 'any substance or combination of substances presented for treating or preventing disease in human beings' (Medicines for Human Use [Marketing Authorisations, etc] Regulations, 1994). The active ingredients in the licensed medicines for head lice currently used in the UK are pharmaceutical grade pesticides belonging to three resistance groups: malathion (organophosphate); phenothrin and permethrin (pyrethroids); and carbaryl (carbamate). Pest populations which acquire resistance to a specific pesticide simultaneously acquire resistance to all pesticides in that chemical group, eg. permethrin resistance confers phenothrin resistance. Carbaryl products became prescription-only medicines (PoM) in January 1996 due to a possible cancer link and may not be prescribed by nurses who have obtained prescribing status. These nurses may only prescribe malathion, phenothrin and permethrin medicines.

The effect of government policy encouraging people towards home health care (DoH, 1992) and concerns about the safety of repeated use of conventional pesticide treatments (eg. Mar, 1995) has led to many unlicensed 'natural' treatments appearing on the market. As part of regulatory action, the MCA issued guidance in February 2000 stating that no product without a licence may mention head lice, nits or infestation, nor can there be any implication that the product is intended to treat these, eg. in a product name, or graphics or by mention of a fine-tooth or nit comb. Licensing is demanded partly because agents capable of killing lice are likely to be potentially toxic to humans. The ruling made an exception for ordinary hair conditioners used to ease the removal of lice and nits with the aid of a fine-tooth comb, which are available as separate products. Any product recommended solely for use as a repellent must not be supplied with a fine-tooth comb and falls under cosmetic regulations or the General Products Safety Regulations (SI 1994 2328). None of these is available on free prescription.

Efficacy

Shampoo formulations (not prescribable on the NHS) are not recommended because the pesticide, diluted by water during the lathering process, is not left on the head long enough to ensure egg-kill. Treatment failure with other formulations, which all claim to kill lice and their eggs in a single application, is a source of increasing frustration (Downs *et al*, 1999; Hill, 1999). To compensate for incomplete egg-kill, the *British National Formulary* (*BNF*) has been suggesting two applications a week apart (ie. day one and day eight) since 1991 (Ibarra, 1998). *Prescribing Nurse Bulletin* (National Prescribing Centre, 1999) adopted this suggestion. Nurses complain it is confusing to give advice that conflicts with the written product instructions (Adair, 2000). Those conversant with the life cycle and behaviour of lice point out that lice emerging soon after the first application may leave the head before day eight, and some eggs may hatch on days nine and ten, so the *BNF* advice is not failsafe. Meanwhile, the MCA does not consider it appropriate for the Licensing Authority to comment on clinical guidelines even though they contradict licensed product instructions.

The first systematic review of clinical efficacy (Vander Stichele *et al*, 1995) found seven trials were of acceptable methodological quality, but the reviewers' criteria did not include checking the hatch rate of treated eggs against untreated eggs after incubation, simulating conditions on the head (Stallbaumer and Ibarra, 1995). Inclusion of this criterion reduces 'adequate trials' to one (Taplin *et al*, 1986), which tested the pyrethroid, permethrin, in a creme rinse formula in Central America, where the head lice population had no history of systematic pesticide exposure. Evidence of the development of resistance to pyrethroids in the UK was also published in 1995 (Burgess *et al*, 1995). Reviewers found insufficient evidence to support the efficacy of carbaryl, corroborating pre-1988 observations made by school nurses. Malathion is also no longer reliable (Downs *et al*, 1999; Hill, 1999). The 1999 Cochrane review could find no contemporary evidence of effectiveness for any of the four pesticides used in the UK (Dodd, 1999).

To put the options fairly to parents, the DoH and CHC have together developed the policy of advising parents to check thoroughly for lice hatching from inadequately treated eggs three to five days after using medication. When hatchlings are found at this stage, parents may choose another pesticide from an alternative resistance group (followed by another check) or commit to correct use of the Bug Buster kit to clear infestation. As with all protocols, if not followed exactly, the Bug Busting method will work by luck rather than design. The failure of vague 'wet combing' undermines confidence in authentic Bug Busting. The Royal College of Nursing (Hancock, 1999) and the Community Practitioners' and Health Visitors' Association (CPHVA, 1999) also aim to offer an informed treatment choice. In contrast, no product carries a warning that lice may have developed resistance to active ingredients, and parents new to the problem tend to learn about treatment failure from bitter experience.

A 'snapshot' randomised, controlled trial (RCT) in North Wales of the 1996 Bug Buster kit (containing the first Bug Buster comb) versus two overnight applications of malathion lotion reported success rates of 38% and 78% respectively (Roberts *et al*,

2000). The result for the Bug Busting method was achieved without initial demonstration and using the more laborious comb (Anon, 2000). Families face multiple episodes of infestation, and exposure of lice to repeatedly applied pesticide promotes resistance, whereas skill at Bug Busting grows with familiarity. No information on sustainability was gathered, although the trial was well-resourced. The 1998 Kit (with an improved comb) is now undergoing independent evaluation in comparison with licensed products used in accordance with the instructions, stating that a single application is sufficient. This RCT, run by the London School of Hygiene and Tropical Medicine, is a three-year project, involving a wide area and data set, including the issue of sustainability.

Safety

All malathion, carbaryl and phenothrin products except shampoo formulas state that they must not be used more than once a week for three consecutive weeks. Although the warnings are product specific, it follows that it is unwise to use any combination of pesticides in excess of this frequency. Special care must be taken with pregnant mothers and women trying to conceive, nursing mothers, infants, and those with multiple chemical sensitivity, who should avoid pesticides as much as possible. The fumes of alcoholic formulas can provoke an asthma attack in susceptible people. They are also flammable.

Conventional pesticide and essential oil ingredients are delivered to hatched lice and their eggs by absorption into the lipids of the outer layer (cuticle) of the insect. Products are designed to be lipophilic in order to release the active ingredients easily into fat. The outer layer of human skin is lipid-saturated. Topical applications of lipophilic formula are therefore drawn through the skin by this fat (Wester and Maibach, 1985). They are applied to the dry scalp for a period ranging from two hours to overnight. During this period evaporation of the vehicle ingredients concentrates the pesticide in the target area. Some penetrating ingredients may cause systemic effects, eg. malathion is immunosuppressive (Rodgers and Ellefson, 1992), terpenoides, derived from tea tree oil are neurotoxic (Downs *et al*, 2000), and carbaryl is also neurotoxic (Maibach *et al*, 1971).

The role of conditioner used in Bug Busting is not parasiticidal. It merely immobilises the lice temporarily by keeping them wet and facilitates their removal with the Bug Buster comb. The time the conditioner is on the head is relatively short, duration of use varying according to the hair type. Typically this is two minutes for short straight hair, or about thirty minutes for tight curly hair. The protocol only requires four such applications in two weeks. Nevertheless, the possibility of adverse effects from conditioner ingredients has been raised by Aston (2000), an advocate of two overnight applications to the dry scalp of malathion or carbaryl lotion a week apart.

For Bug Busting, conditioner is applied to a wet scalp so any oily molecules are not offered much purchase. Combing begins immediately after application which spreads the conditioner down the hair length. With each sweep of the comb some is removed, and then the remainder is thoroughly rinsed off. Bug Busting always uses 'wash-out' conditioner, but 'leave-in' conditioner also contains the ingredients that concern Aston. Neither variety carries warnings against exceeding a certain frequency of use or application time. In the case of individual localised reactions to conditioner — such as skin irritation — this can be avoided by switching to another brand.

Quality

Two trials, where trained hairdressers (Bingham *et al*, 2000) or nurses (Plastow *et al*, 2000) achieved poor results with pesticide products, suggest that parental non-compliance with treatment instructions is not necessarily the reason for treatment failure. The criteria applied before granting a licence are not in the public domain and post-marketing vigilance does not monitor resistance development. There are calls for National Institute for Clinical Excellence assessment.

Cost

A single application of a licensed parasiticidal product costs approximately £2.15 (NHS) or £3.79 (OTC). The Bug Buster Kit, which is reusable, costs £5.95 including postage and packing (*Table 3.2*).

Table 3.2: Resources
Licensed products that nurses may prescribe are listed in the *Nurse Prescribers' Formulary* at N17–18.
The leaflet, *The Prevention and Treatment of Head Lice* (DoH, 2000b) is available free to schools and health professionals in the UK from: Department of Health, PO Box 777, London SE1 6XH; fax: 01623 724 524. It is available in English and ten ethnic languages.
The 'Stafford Group' video *Head louse control from the classroom to the community!* (SSL International, 1999) is free to healthcare professionals. Tel: 01565 624000.
Bug Buster Kits and a demonstration video of the Bug Busting method can be purchased from Community Hygiene Concern, by phone or online. Tel: 020 7686 4321; internet: http://www.nits.net/bugbusting
Bug Buster Help Line: 020 7686 4321.

Prescribing policy

Some areas of the UK have adopted the 'Stafford Group' (Aston *et al*, 1998) recommendations for six consecutive applications, a week apart (two applications of a product from each pesticide group) for persistent cases. Bug Busting may be used as a detection method, but is reserved as a last resort, rather than a means of introducing parental self-reliance in treatment. However, any nurse prescribing raises issues of accountability and patient safety (Baird, 2000). Nurses with prescriber status should follow local policy guidelines, but have a duty to monitor outcomes. This can be done by supervising adequate checking three to five days after prescribed medication, or a check on day seventeen after initiating Bug Busting.

Conclusion

According to published evidence, in North Wales one child in four or five treated with malathion suffers treatment failure (Roberts *et al*, 2000) and in Bristol and Bath pyrethroids are less than 20% effective (Downs *et al*, 1999). Resistance can increase 100-fold in the period between completing a study and publication (Hill, 2000). Expenditure on medication and professional time is likely to escalate in a deteriorating scenario unless prescribing nurses seek to ensure that clinical governance prevails.

The work of Community Hygiene Concern on head lice is currently part-funded by the Department of Health and the National Lottery Charities Board.

Key Points

❃ Do not prescribe chemotherapy for head lice without confirming diagnosis accurately.

❃ Bug Busting wet combing is a reliable detection method. Parents should be encouraged to learn the skill using the correct comb and instructions.

❃ Nurses with prescribing status may prescribe malathion and pyrethroids, but they have a high failure rate.

❃ Alternatively, commitment to systematic Bug Busting can clear an infestation.

❃ Prescribing nurses should follow local policy guidelines, monitor outcomes and seek to ensure that clinical governance prevails.

References

Adair M (2000) The head louse debate. *Prof Care Mother Child* **10**(4): 106

Anon (2000) Head lice: the gentle skill of Bug Busting. *Shared Wisdom* **5**: 4–5

Aston R, Duggal H, Simpson J, advised by Burgess I ('Stafford Group') (1998) *Head Lice. Report for Consultants in Communicable Disease Control (CCDCs)* http://www.fam-english.demon.co.uk/phmeghl.htm

Aston R (2000) The head louse debate. *Prof Care Mother Child* **10**(5): 134–5

Baird A (2000) Crown II: the implications of nurse prescribing for practice nursing. *Br J Community Nurs* **5**(9): 454–61

Bingham P, Kirk S, Hill N, Figueroa J (2000) The methodology and operation of a pilot randomized control trial of the effectiveness of the Bug Busting method against a single application insecticide product for head louse treatment. *Public Health* **114**: 265–8

Burgess IF, Pcock S, Brown CM, Kaufman J (1995) Head lice resistant to pyrethroid insecticides in Britain. *Br Med J* **311**: 752

Chemist & Druggist (1995) Some lousy facts. *Chemist & Druggist* **244**: 124

Community Practitioners' and Health Visitors' Association (1999) *Head lice report has 'major flaws', says CPHVA.* Press release. CPHVA, London 14 July

De Maeseneer J, Blokland I, Willems S, Vander Stichele R, Meersschaut F (2000) Wet combing versus traditional scalp inspection to detect head lice in schoolchildren: observational study. *Br Med J* **321**: 1187–8

Department of Health (1992) *Virginia Bottomley outlines way forward on controlling increase in NHS drugs bill.* Press release. H92/430, 1 Dec

Department of Health (2000a) *A Health Service of All the Talents: Developing the NHS Workforce.* The Stationery Office, London

Department of Health (2000b) *The Prevention and Treatment of Head Lice.* Leaflet (LO9/001 10860 1P 50k TR SA Feb 00). DoH, London

Dodd CS (1999) *Interventions for the treatment of head lice*. Cochrane Database of Systematic Reviews. The Cochrane Library. Cochrane Collaboration. Update Software, Oxford

Downs AMR, Stafford KA, Harvey I, Coles GC (1999) Evidence for double resistance to permethrin and malathion in head lice. *Br J Dermatol* **141**: 508–11

Downs AMR, Stafford KA, Coles GC (2000) Monoterpenoids and tetralin as pediculocides. *Acta Derm Venereol* **1**: 69–70

Hall DMB, Holroyd E, Ibarra J (1995) *GP receptionist involvement in the management of head infestation*. Unpublished survey results

Hancock C (1999) *Royal College of Nursing position on the treatment of head lice*. http://www.chc.org/ noticeboard.html

Hase A (1931) Siphunculata; Anoplura; Aptera. Lause. *Biologie der Tiere Deutschlands* **34**: 1–58

Hill N (1999) Why are we failing to control head lice with insecticides? Proceedings of the 3rd International Conference on Urban Pests 1999: 635

Hill N (2000) Treatment of head lice. *Lancet* **356**: 2007

Ibarra J (1998) Pesticides for topical use. In: Figueroa J, Hall S, Ibarra J, eds. *Primary Health Care Guide to Common UK Parasitic Diseases*. Community Hygiene Concern, London: 37–45

Ibarra J, Fry F, Brooks P, Scott E, Lesley Smith J (2000) Interim Report: Study comparing visual inspection at school with use of the 1998 Bug Buster Kit at home for the detection of head infestation. *Shared Wisdom* **5**: 10–11

Maibach HI, Fledman RJ, Milby TH, Serat WF (1971) Regional variation in percutaneous penetration in man. *Arch Environ Health* **23**: 208–11

Mar M (1995) Head lice: remedial advice. *Hansard* 27 Nov: 454–6

Mellanby K (1942) Natural population of the head louse (Pediculus humanus capitis: Anoplura) on infected children in England. *Parasitology* **34**: 180–4

National Prescribing Centre (1999) Management of head louse infection. *Prescrib Nurse Bull* **1**(4): 13–16

Owen CM (1982) Too much nit-picking? *Nurs Times* **78**: 632–34

Plastow L, Luthra M, Powell R, Marshall M, Wright J, Russell D (2000) A randomised controlled trial comparing the effectiveness of traditional head lice treatments with the bug busting method in the management of head lice infestation. Presentation to Clinical Excellence 2000, Harrogate: 30 Nov

Purcell S (1998) Practical ways with parasites. *Chemist & Druggist* **250**: 14–16

Roberts RJ, Casey D, Morgan DA, Petrovic M (2000) Comparison of wet combing with malathion for treatment of head lice in the UK: a pragmatic randomised controlled trial. *Lancet* **356**: 540–4

Rodgers K, Ellefson D (1992) Mechanism of the modulation of murine peritoneal cell function and mast cell degranulation by low doses of malathion. *Agents Actions* **35**: 57–63

Stallbaumer M, Ibarra J (1995) Counting head lice by visual inspection flaws trials' results. *Br Med J* **311**: 1369

Taplin D, Meinking TL, Castillero PM and Sanchez R (1986) Permethrin 1% creme rinse for the treatment of *Pediculus humanus var capitis* infestation. *Pediatr Dermatol* **3**: 344–8

Vander Stichele RH, Dezeure EM, Bogaert MG (1995) Systematic review of clinical efficacy of topical treatments for head lice. *Br Med J* **311**: 604–8

Wester RC, Maibach HI (1985) In vivo percutaneous absorption and decontamination of pesticides in humans. *J Toxicol Environ Health* **16**(1): 25–37

4

Threadworms: a starting point for family hygiene

Joanna Ibarra

Owing to the embarrassing anal itch caused by threadworm infection, some sufferers feel they cannot even mention the problem to their doctor. Community nurses, often regarded as a more approachable source of support, will also be able to prescribe medication if they have prescribing status. With an adequate understanding of the complaint, they can offer a choice of treatment options, mechanical removal or drugs, necessarily backed by the appropriate personal and environmental hygiene measures. The starting point for relevant hygiene is cheerful good practice in hand washing at home and school, which is also key to preventing the spread of many other more serious infections. Implementation is of basic importance and should form part of any of the current initiatives from Sure Start to Healthy Schools.

It is reasonable to believe that threadworm infection (enterobiasis) has been endemic in the UK since humans first appeared on these islands. *Enterobius vermicularis* is the commonest parasitic worm of humans, endemic in all human populations to varying degrees. A small nematode, it has evolved the capacity to successfully parasitise *Homo sapiens*, but no other species. There was once open recognition of the intensely uncomfortable itching anus characteristic of threadworm infection, as graphically described by Phaer in 1544: 'The excedyng ytche in the fundament' (Phaer, 1544). Now, it is regarded as an unmentionable embarrassment and confidential treatment is sought. Today, sufferers may feel unable to talk about worms even with their doctor. Nurses present a more approachable image and are more likely to be consulted.

Nurses take the lead in control

Since 1999, a suitably qualified nurse with prescribing status may prescribe drug treatment for threadworms and so is enabled to take full responsibility for managing patients with enterobiasis. It can be argued that a prescribing nurse is the most appropriate member of the primary care team to manage patients with these parasites. One-off infections are often treated with medicines purchased in retail pharmacies. However when recurrence is the problem, patients are prompted to seek sympathy and advice from a nurse. It is important that the nurse's understanding of the complaint is adequate, and that treatment of the individual is couched within family and community action geared to prevention, or recurrence will probably continue.

Transmission

Mature threadworms do not pass from person to person. Threadworm infection is caught by swallowing, or inhaling and then swallowing, the egg. The female worm lays her eggs in the perianal folds and they are thence transferred on scratching fingers directly to the mouth, or indirectly after they have been shed into the environment as an infected person moves about. They settle as dust in the home and communal toilet areas where infected people lower their underwear. They can end up on toothbrushes, toys and food. In cool, moist conditions they can survive several days, possibly some weeks (Nolan and Reardon, 1939; Muller, 1975) (*Box 4.1*).

A common, generally benign, complaint

Many people, especially children, catch threadworms. At least 30% of children will have them in their early years. Studies that examine incidence over a period of time are very limited. Ibarra (1989) surveyed parents of children attending a single primary school by confidential questionnaire. They were asked to recall episodes of threadworm in the family over the past year. Nearly half those who reported cases had experienced repeated infection, one person having six episodes in the year. Calls to the charity Community

Hygiene Concern (CHC) help line from 1989 onwards confirm that recurrence is a major problem.

Parents need reassurance that threadworms are generally harmless. Unfortunately, enormous unnecessary distress has been caused by various publications and web-site entries erroneously suggesting that threadworms can be caught from soil. This has coincided with rising awareness that infection with the eggs of dog and cat roundworm (*Toxocara sp.*) is picked up from contaminated soil, and can cause blindness in human. Nurses have an important contribution to make in clearing up this confusion.

Box 4.1: Threadworm life cycle and behaviour

Threadworm or pinworm (*Enterobius vermicularis*) is a small, white, thread-like worm between 2 and 13mm long. The male reaches a maximum of 5mm.

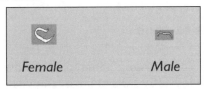

Female   Male

* Female threadworms produce large numbers of tiny eggs (50 x 20 μm), invisible to the naked eye. The female lays these eggs outside the anus in the perianal folds, or in girls, around and inside the vagina or urethra, when the host is still, such as asleep; inactivity of the host promotes migration of the female to the anus.

* The eggs are laid in a sticky secretion which can cause intense itching and provokes scratching by the host. Later the eggs lose their stickiness and float, settling as dust indoors. In cool, moist conditions they take some time to die. Eggs collecting in the home and community toilet areas where infected people lower their underwear are a major environmental source of infection.

* Infection begins by swallowing the eggs or inhaling and then swallowing them. The eggs hatch in the duodenum. The worms develop by moulting three times, reaching maturity in the intestine, usually in two weeks, occasionally longer. When adult, the male fertilises the female, is expelled in the stools and dies. The female dies after depositing her eggs; she often bursts in the process.

* Re-infection may occur after scratching as when children suck contaminated fingers. Eggs lodge easily under finger nails.

* Additionally some eggs hatch after four hours on the body surface, whereupon the larvae migrate into the caecum via the anus (retrofection or retroinfection). These larvae appear to take longer to complete their life cycle than worms hatching from swallowed eggs.

* The threadworm is a human parasite which does not infect pets.

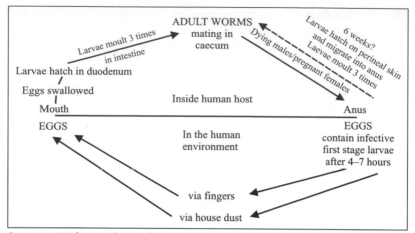

Sources: Nolan and Reardon, 1939; Schuffner and Swellengrebel, 1949; Muller 1975, 1979; Beaver *et al*, 1984

Preparing parents to cope

Tactfully raising awareness among parents of threadworm infection is a responsibility that logically falls to the health visitor, since it can be a problem in babies. A parent may observe the thread-like female emerging from a child's anus after a bath. The males can sometimes be seen moving on the surface of the stools, and are particularly noticeable when a child is in nappies. Parents should be advised to gently remove a suspect worm from the anus with a cotton bud and a drop of vegetable oil or baby lotion. If there is any doubt the sample should be placed in a plastic bag and sealed to show to a community nurse.

There are circumstances when a check for threadworms is indicated, although the characteristic anal itching is absent:

❖ Bedwetting in a normally dry child should immediately raise a high index of suspicion (Jacobs, 1942). There is a good case for routinely checking all new patients attending enuresis clinics.

❖ In girls with vaginal discharge or irritation a check for threadworm infection should also be routinely made (Pierce and Hart, 1992). The propensity of the female worm to migrate to the vagina or urethra in girls after emerging from the anus and to lay her eggs there instead of the perianal folds can cause serious ill health. The worm often carries *Escherichia coli* and other faecal organisms with it (Simon, 1974; O'Brien, 1995).

❖ If one member of the family has threadworms, the other members should check for infection.

❖ Children should be checked when warning of an outbreak at parents' or baby/toddler groups, nursery or school is issued.

How to check for threadworms

Depending on sight of the males in the stools is fairly unreliable. Evidence of the female is more easily found by examination of the anal area when a child is at rest, taking care not to make the child uncomfortable. Worms can be caught leaving the anus using wide hypoallergenic tape pressed gently right against the anus. The tape should be applied as a child goes to bed and closely fitting underpants put on to keep it in place. The tape is then gently removed in the morning. Alternatively, a large blob of petroleum jelly (or petroleum jelly substitute) can be applied to the anus on retiring, also with closely fitting pants over, carefully wiped off with tissue first thing in the morning and examined for the presence of worms. These home methods do not require special equipment since the worm is recognisable with the naked eye. However, to confirm diagnosis the sample should be placed in a plastic bag and sealed to show to the health visitor.

More costly in professional time is diagnosis made by taking an anal swab. This should be done early in the day before the patient washes the anal area after rising. Clear cellophane tape is applied to the anus to pick up any threadworm eggs, pressed on a slide and examined for eggs under a microscope. It may be necessary to make tests four mornings in a row to be certain, because most infections are light. Analysis of stool samples should only be considered if other worm infections are suspected since threadworm eggs often do not appear in the stools.

Treatment options

There are two treatment options; mechanical removal and drugs. Treatment of an individual should be preceded with a check of close contacts and treatment of all infected people in the same household should then be initiated simultaneously. Whichever treatment option is chosen it is essential to combine it with measures of personal and environmental hygiene. This prevents additional infections and reinfection within the household.

Mechanical removal

The methods described here have been used successfully by some people reporting to CHC. These people are unable or unwilling to take medication (eg. pregnant/nursing mothers). The measures suggested must be applied for a minimum of two weeks to remove all females maturing from eggs swallowed before the commencement of treatment. An individual's infection ends naturally when all males are expelled after mating and all females have died after laying their eggs. This cycle usually takes two to three weeks to complete, but completion of the cycle depends on ceasing to ingest new eggs and preventing any retroinfection. The first objective is achieved by means of adequate personal and environmental hygiene; retro-infection can be prevented by applying tape or jelly at night, washing or wet-wiping the perianal area first thing in the morning and at three-hourly intervals during the day (since it takes at least four hours for infective first stage larvae to develop after egg-laying). Use soft toilet paper moistened with plain vegetable oil or baby lotion as wet-wipes because they can be flushed safely after use.

If a baby is in nappies, all eggs and worms will be caught in the nappy and the eggs prevented from contaminating the home. Be careful to cleanse the bottom gently but thoroughly at nappy changes. Make changes at least every three hours to prevent any return through the anus of worms hatching in the nappy.

Drug (anthelmintic) treatment

Currently there are two active ingredients in use for threadworms in the UK, mebendazole and piperazine, in various presentations (*Table 4.1*). They are also used to treat infection with human roundworm (*Ascaris lumbricoides*) and other more serious infections. A nurse with prescribing status may prescribe parasiticidal medicines for threadworms but not for other worm infections, which require medical consultation. In principle, pregnant women wishing to take drug treatment for threadworms should be referred for medical advice.

Children under two years old may be treated with mebendazole, and under one with piperazine on medical advice only.

Medicines containing senna should be avoided for young children due to their dehydrating effect; a course of piperazine citrate elixir may be the most suitable choice. Medication of children under two years old, and pregnant and nursing mothers is inadvisable. Pregnant mothers should be assured that no harm will come to a child born while the mother has threadworms (Pietroni and Davidson, 1996). Breastfed babies are less likely to catch threadworms and more easily get over threadworms than bottle fed babies (Romanenko *et al*, 1997).

Mebendazole is, on balance, safer than piperazine (Cook, 1994) but is not licensed for children under two years old, pregnant and nursing mothers. Mebendazole acts mainly in the gut with very little intestinal absorption and most of the drug is excreted in the stools (Nathan, 1997). Systemic side-effects are probably more common with piperazine, including, rarely, muscular inco-ordination ('worm wobble') (Prescribing Nurse Bulletin, 1999). It would be most unwise to use head lice and threadworm medication simultaneously; it could lead to pesticide overdose.

Neither piperazine nor mebendazole kills recently swallowed eggs, and piperazine does not affect larval worms, so a second dose, or course of treatment, at fourteen days is often required. Mebendazole products do not state this, merely suggesting that repeat treatment at two to three weeks will be necessary for re-infection. During the period of thirteen days after a dose of either, all egg-laying should cease. However, adequate personal and environmental hygiene remains important to avoid re-infection from eggs already in clothes, bedding etc.

Reducing the spread of eggs

Appropriate personal and environmental hygiene are the best defence against threadworm infection and reinfection.

Table 4.1: Threadworm treatments available for nurse prescription and over the counter (OTC) at a pharmacy

Medicine/ manufacturer	Active ingredients	Product instructions	Product warnings	Comments
Ovex Janssen-Cilag	100mg mebendazole per tablet	Single tablet dose (chewed or swallowed whole) for adults and children aged two and over	• Not to be taken by children under two, pregnant or nursing mothers, or in combination with cimetidine (for stomach acidity) except on medical advice • Minor side-effects such as mild, short-lived stomach ache, diarrhoea or allergic reactions — rashes, shortness of breath or itching — are rare. Report any other side-effects to doctor or pharmacist	• Product leaflet mistakenly advises that threadworm eggs can be picked up in garden soil or on unwashed vegetables and salads • It is advisable to report all unwanted effects to doctor or pharmacist
Pripsen sachets SSL international	4gm piperazine phosphate and 300mg senna per sachet	Dual dose, second sachet taken 14 days after first sachet. Sachet contents stirred into water or milk and drunk immediately. Children aged 1–6 years to be restricted to 5ml of the powder	• Not to be taken by pregnant mothers. If taken by nursing mothers stop breastfeeding for 8 hours and throw away expressed milk • Not to be taken by infants up to one-year-old without medical advice • Not to be taken by sufferers of epilepsy, kidney or liver disease, those allergic to piperazine or in conjunction with sedatives, antidepressants, diuretics, cardiac glycosides, 'adrenocorticosteroid preparations' without medical consultation • Uncommon side-effects, listed as rash, itching, wheezing, gastrointestinal upsets, dizziness, weakness and aching muscles, should be reported to your doctor straight away	• It is not practical for many mothers to suddenly express breast milk instead of feeding • Senna can cause severe dehydration in young children • When consulted SSL International explained that 'adrenocortico-steroid preparations' includes asthma inhalers and eczema ointments and some rheumatoid arthritis treatments. The product leaflet does not give this information in a widely comprehensible way

Table 4.1: cont.

		Comments
Pripsen elixir SSL international	750mg piperazine citrate per 5ml. Product is 96% alcohol	Taken by 5ml spoonful daily for 7 days, followed by 7 days rest and then another 7 days daily administration. Adults and children over 12 years 3x5ml; 7–12 years 2x5ml; 4–6 years, 1.5x5ml; 1–3 years, 1x5ml	• Not to be taken by those sensitive to the ingredients, by sufferers of epilepsy, kidney or liver disease • Not to be taken by pregnant or nursing mothers • Not for use in children under one year without medical advice • Not to be taken in conjunction with 'phenothiazine products' without consultation with doctor or pharmacist • Report possible undesirable effects of nausea, vomiting, diarrhoea, stomach pains, headaches and rashes to doctor or pharmacist, having discontinued use immediately	• The warning about mixing with 'phenothiazine products' is unlikely to be understandable by the general public
Pripsen tablets SSL international	100mg mebendazole per tablet	Single table dose (chewed or swallowed with water) for adults and children aged two and over	• Not to be taken by pregnant or nursing mothers, or those sensitive to the ingredients without medical advice. Not recommended for children under two years • Undesirable effects reported after use are rare abdominal pain and diarrhoea, or hyper-sensibility reactions, rashes, redness, itchiness. Report any other reaction to doctor or pharmacist	• It is advisable to report all unwanted effects to doctor or pharmacist

Source: All information other than 'Comments' is drawn from product packaging
NB: A mebendazole suspension (Vermox, Janssen-Cilag) is available for prescription but not OTC; Boots sell their own brand of mebendazole tables, available OTC

Personal hygiene

The key personal hygiene measure is adequate hand washing after going to the toilet and before preparing and eating food. It is not surprising, therefore, that children are particularly vulnerable to threadworms while they are learning these skills. Children should be helped by keeping their nails short and providing clean underpants each day, or more often if necessary.

Parents need support in teaching their children how to go to the toilet hygienically and wash their hands properly. This provides protection against threadworms and a wide range of other infections, not least gastroenteritis. Good habits cheerfully established in the early years will set a child up for life (*Table 4.2*). Playgroups, drop-in centres, nurseries and primary schools should be encouraged to supervise hand washing until children are seven years old. This is an issue of basic importance which should be raised at group and school management meetings. Implementation of an adequate hand washing programme through any of the current initiatives — Healthy Living Centres, Sure Start, Early Years Development and Childcare Partnership, Health Action Zones, New Deal for Lone Parents and Healthy Schools Initiative — making use of trained volunteers, would be progress indeed.

Environmental hygiene

Raising hand washing standards is, however, only part of the issue. It needs to be coupled with environmental hygiene designed to remove threadworm eggs from the home and community facilities. At home on the first day of personal treatment, whether using medicines or not, sleepwear, bedlinen, towels, and cuddly toys should be changed and washed. Washing can be done at normal temperatures as long as it is well rinsed. The house should be vacuum cleaned and dusted thoroughly. Toothbrushes should be rinsed well before use.

Co-ordination of a draconian assault on accumulated eggs with the first day of treatment allows a family to relax back into normal cleaning thereafter, a more practical approach for busy families than the oft-proposed six-week stint. Moreover, obsessive, rather than automatic well-targeted hygiene, should not be encouraged.

Gatherer (1978) established that up to 90% of infected individuals do not feel any anal irritation; as a result they are unaware that they are spreading threadworm eggs. This causes misery to other families sharing the use of community facilities who suffer symptoms whenever they catch threadworms. Whatever care they take at home and with their own hygiene, they are not fully protected from the reservoir of viable eggs which accumulates elsewhere if cleaning is inadequate. It must be explained that although bleach and disinfectants may be effective against viral and bacterial infections, they are useless against worm eggs. Heating dries out and kills worm eggs, and good ventilation will assist their dispersal but many toilet areas are not heated or well ventilated. A regular routine of physical removal by vacuum cleaning and/or lifting with damp paper is necessary. Community nurses have a key role to play in disseminating this information and encouraging the community to 'make the best' of their facilities, where the correct hygiene strategy can raise their quality.

Table 4.2: Hand washing check list

At home	Teach children to wipe the bottom with one hand and to turn on the tap for washing afterwards with the other hand. In girls always wipe from the front in a backwards direction, away from the vagina.
	Show children how to wash with soap to loosen dirt and then use running water to rinse, so the force of the water carries away the dirt. When the risk of scalding water cannot be eliminated, teach children to use the cold tap.
	Show children how to judge whether washing has been efficient by checking the towel after drying — dirt or soap stains should not come off on the towel.
At parent and toddler groups, playgroups and nurseries	Make sure help is at hand (with respect for privacy) when children need to use the toilet. It may involve young children in a lot of thought and they can be easily distracted if rushed. Hand washing should be supervised afterwards.
	Do not expect anti-bacterial washes to safeguard children from infections they could pickup if playing with toilets or drains.
	Do not substitute bowls of rinsing water, which become reservoirs of infection, for hand washing before eating.
At primary school	Appoint soap and towel monitors — at playtime these should be adult, during class time pupils can become keepers of the soap on a rotational basis as part of learning about personal hygiene.
Everywhere	Promote enthusiasm for personal hygiene; guard against turning hand washing into a chore.
	Discourage intermittent snacking and supervise hand washing before regular meals, as part of healthy eating.

Conclusion

The minority of families who are conscious of their repeated threadworm infections is in danger of feeling socially humiliated in a society which shuns those who harbour personal parasites. Community nurses have the opportunity to focus attention on specific remedial measures within a broad spectrum of healthy living projects where they inform and contribute to policy-making decisions. Implementation brings hygiene benefits and well-being to the general community far beyond relief to families and individuals with recurring threadworm problems.

> *The work of CHC Threadworm Help Line Counsellor, Pauline Shimell, has provided significant insights into the management of enterobiasis, which are freely drawn on in this chapter. The CHC project, Community Action against Parasites, is part funded by the Department of Health.*

Key Points

❊ Threadworm infection is widespread and commonly recurs, an acute embarrassment to those who experience the characteristic anal itching.

❊ It is important that the treatment of the individual is couched within family and community action geared to prevention of new and recurring cases.

❊ Community nurses are well placed to take the lead in implementing personal and environmental hygiene measures which protect against threadworms and a wide range of other infections, not least gastroenteritis.

References

Beaver PC, Jung RC, Cupp EW (1984) Oxyuroidea and Ascaridoidea. In: *Clinical Parasitology*, 9th edn. Lea and Febiger, Philadelphia: 302–6

Cook GE (1994) Enterobius vermicularis infection. *Gut* **35**: 1159–62

Gatherer A (1978) A common problem. *Nursing Times Community Outlook* **74**: 303–4

Ibarra J (1989) Towards a viable approach to the threadworm problem. *Health at School* **5**: 54–7

Jacobs AH (1942) Enterobiasis in children: incidence, symptomatology and diagnosis with a simplified Scotch cellulose tape technique. *J Paediatr* **21**: 497–503

Muller R (1975) Enterobius vermicularis. In: *Worms and Disease: a manual of medical helminthology.* Heinemann Medical, London: 89–91

Muller R (1979) Nematodes. In: RJ Donaldson, ed. *Parasites and Western Man.* MTP Press, Lancaster: 78–113

Nathan A (1997) A non-prescription medicines formulary no. 13. *Anthelmintics. Pharm J* **258**: 770–1

Nolan MO, Reardon L (1939) Studies on oxyuriasis. XX. The distribution of the ova of *Enterobius vermicularis* in household dust. *J Parasitol* **25**: 173–7

O'Brien TJ (1995) Paediatric vulvovaginitis. *Aust J Dermatol* **36**: 216–18

Phaer T (1544) *The Boke of Children*: xiii

Pierce AM, Hart CA (1992) Vulvovaginitis: causes and management. *Arch Dis Child* **67**: 509–12

Pietroni M, Davidson R (1996) Treatments for worm infections seen in the UK. *Prescriber* **7**: 33–44

Prescribing Nurse Bulletin (1999) Threadworms. *Prescrib Nurse Bull* **1**: 11–12

Romanenko HA, Serglev VP, Chernyshenko AI *et al* (1997) New approaches to the eradication of enterobiasis in children. *Med Parazitol Mosk* **1**: 3–5

Schuffner W, Swellengrebel NH (1949) Retrofection in oxyuriasis. A newly discovered mode of infection with Enterobius vermicularis. *J Parasitol* **35**: 138–46

Simon RD (1974) Pinworm infestation and urinary tract infection in young girls. *Am J Dis Child* **128**: 21–2

5

Record keeping and nurse prescribing: an issue of concern?

Xena Dion

As options are explored by the NHS Executive to extend nurse prescribing in terms of expanding the Nurse Prescribers' Formulary and widening the groups of nurses eligible to train to prescribe, issues surrounding record keeping in the community need to be revisited in order to safeguard professional integrity. Prescribing nurses in the community face barriers to accurate and adequate record keeping when access to all patients' records is not permitted and/or time constraints and extra travelling impede the process, potentially threatening the safety of the patient. Until information technology provides the answer to safe and effective use of shared patient records, nurses who prescribe any treatments need to ensure they share full access to all patients' notes.

The publication of new plans and a guide for implementation to extend nurse prescribing (DoH, 2002) confirms the expectations of both an expansion of the groups of nurses eligible to prescribe and a widely extended formulary of drugs from which certain nurses may prescribe. Exciting though this may be for nurses who look forward to using prescribing to enhance patient care and to pursue professional self-development, the implications to practice in terms of professional accountability and responsibility are formidable. The Government's justification for extending nurse prescribing is to improve patient care by providing faster and more efficient access to medicines and to make full use of nursing skills. Foremost in the verification of good practice and acknowledgement of accountability, lies adequate and accurate record keeping. In the community, however, the very arena from which nurse prescribing stemmed, accessing patient's notes to record prescribing information and reported time pressures, presents nurses with complications and barriers that potentially threaten their professional integrity.

Accountability and record keeping

Professional accountability is not new to nurses and prescribing is only another extension of that in a time of considerable expansion of roles and responsibilities, demanding the same skills of professional assessment, judgement and decision making used in other areas of practice (Cresswell, 1998). There is no ambiguity in where the responsibility and accountability lies behind nurse prescribing. The United Kingdom Central Council for Nursing, Midwifery and Health Visiting (UKCC) (1992a, b) stated clearly that nurses are personally responsible for ensuring they are working within their level of competence and that they recognise their limitations in practice. Accountability is laid directly at the feet of nurses themselves in all areas of practice:

> *As a registered nurse, midwife or health visitor you are personally accountable for your practice...*

> (UKCC, 1992b)

The law itself clarifies any doubt regarding accountability when prescribing, by stating that whoever signs the prescription is legally responsible (Cresswell, 1998). Although Dimond (2000a) specifies that further legislation will be necessary to fully implement the proposals put forward in the Crown Review (DoH, 1999), the review team state clearly that individual practitioners, 'are the prime custodians of safe and effective clinical practice, including prescribing'. There is no doubt that whatever circumstances arise surrounding nurse prescribing, the individual nurses, and no-one else, is responsible and accountable for their actions.

Patient safety and record keeping

Accountability goes hand-in-hand with taking 'ownership' of professional actions by making a personally signed, permanent record of them. Adequate and accurate record keeping reflects good, safe practice, underpinned by effective communication with other people involved in a person's care. This concept is clearly reinforced in the first Crown Report on nurse prescribing (DoH, 1989), which stated:

> *... the acceptance of prescribing responsibility brings an implicit requirement for the clear and unambiguous recording of information, and for that information to be shared between nurse and doctor and any other healthcare professional involved in the patient's care.*

Efficient record keeping is essentially designed to help protect the welfare of patients (UKCC, 1998) and to promote quality of care for them (Dimond, 2000b). Accurate and adequate completion of patient records provides all professionals involved in a patient's care with the information they need to give continuity of care and practice safely, by avoiding the repeated prescribing of ineffective or harmful therapies (Smallman, 1999).

The current *Nurse Prescribers' Formulary* (*NPF*) contains a myriad of drugs and therapies that potentially can be harmful as well as remedial. The manufacturer's information that accompanies most of the drugs and therapies listed, as well as information provided in the *NPF*, clearly state the possible harm or discomfort that the substances can cause to the patient if either an allergic reaction occurs or if they are prescribed wrongly. If the prescribing event is not recorded in all relevant records, information is inadequate for the next practitioner who may inadvertently prescribe the same harmful agent again and/or repeat the same strength/dose of medication.

Adequate record keeping when prescribing any substance or therapy is essential to the actual well-being of the patient. It is not professionally appropriate or sufficient to rely on patients themselves to remember what they have previously been prescribed or what substances exactly they reacted to. Fragmented record keeping, therefore, potentially compromises the safety of the patient; a large number of clinical negligence cases are caused by failure in the communication process, which could be avoided by accurate record keeping (Tingle, 1998).

Safeguarding the nurse

Maintaining accurate records within the context of nurse prescribing is not just about ensuring quality care and safe practice towards the patient. It is essential as a safeguard for the prescribing nurse in 'proving' professional ability and safe prescribing practice. Nurses should take heed of advice given to doctors when prescribing, that the maintaining of appropriate records, written contemporaneously, is not only considered good practice, but is the best way of challenging unjustified allegations against their practice (Laurence *et al*, 1997). If there is any complaint or cause for concern about the patient's care, the relevant records will be required to carry out an appropriate investigation. Dimond (2000b) makes a formidable list of people who may view those records during such an investigation. This includes review panels, coroners, police, ombudsmen, health authorities and/or trust members and lawyers. The list in itself should act as a grave reminder to nurses who are prescribing, that records must always satisfy legal requirements. Young (1995) specifies that in order to do so, records must be legible; permanent; accurately dated, timed and signed; factual; comprehensive and completed contemporaneously. In addition they should not contain inappropriate information, abbreviations, jargon, errors or alterations. The most common faults by nurses in record keeping are not fulfilling these simple criteria (Dimond, 2000b).

By ensuring they are working within specified guidelines (UKCC, 1992a, b) and that their record keeping satisfies legal requirements, nurses are well placed to safeguard their professional integrity. Yet, despite the fact that litigation against the NHS is increasing (Tingle, 1998), Anderson (2000) claims that, 'nursing documentation is neither done well nor is it popular with nurses' even with increasing emphasis on the matter.

Nurses' ambivalence towards record keeping was investigated by Howse and Bailey (1992) who found several reasons why nurses did not record information adequately, including lack of confidence and/or ability to express themselves in writing, and time pressures. As the practice of prescribing by nurses increases, the demand for health professionals to share information regarding a patient's care and the need for nurses to safeguard themselves against potential litigation also increases. There has never been a more important time for all nurses in primary care to scrutinise their record-keeping practice and make improvements where necessary.

Barriers to shared record keeping

Barriers to sharing accurate and adequate recorded information on patient care appear in several guises. In addition to nurses' individual shortcomings, ambivalence and lack of value of record keeping, despite the importance attached to it (Toms, 1992), the process presents several challenges to them in terms of physical access. While prescribing nurses may well be fully aware of the importance of record keeping in theory and that, 'poor records mean a poor defence and no records means no defence!' (Tingle, 1998), in practice the reality is that recording information in all the appropriate patient records is not always easy or even possible. The Clinical Systems Group of the DoH produced a report (DoH, 1998) highlighting the difficulties members of the primary healthcare team, not employed by the practice (namely district nurses, health visitors and community mental health nurses) have in accessing patient records to obtain or enter information. Clark and Mooney (1999) suggest that only a small number of general practices allow or encourage community nurses to use the practice record system, and that this limited step is not enough to promote a fully integrated approach to patient care. With increasing collaboration between health professionals to address the Government's agenda in primary care (DoH, 1997) through primary care groups and trusts, it is possible that a more cooperative attitude is spreading regarding nurses' access to patient medical records. If this does not happen, nurses who are prescribing and who do not have access to patients' medical notes are well-placed to argue their case that, in the interest of patient safety, they must access medical records to obtain and enter information.

Although formal research has yet to be published on the realities of nurse prescribing, and record keeping specifically, time pressures are perceived to be a problem (Howse and Bailey, 1992). This may be particularly so for community practitioners in rural areas who may be covering more than one GP practice and where distances are considerable. But if time pressures are a real issue, barriers can be overcome, as not all information necessarily has to be recorded in all patient notes. In their nurse prescribing pilot scheme, Berry and Hurst (1999) reached an agreement with their employing trust and practice GPs to save time by not recording all prescribing activity in all patient notes. They agreed that all systemic medicines they prescribed would be recorded in the GP's patient notes in addition to nursing records, but wound products/dressings and appliances would only have to be recorded on patient-held records kept in the patients' homes. The agreement, while saving time for nurses and acknowledging their autonomy in practice in wound management, also demonstrates the need to accept all systemic medicines that nurses can prescribe as significant enough to record in patients' medical records. This not only underpins safe practice, but also lays down good foundations in prescribing practice in preparation for working with an extended formulary where the need for information between professionals grows with the number of drugs nurses will be able to prescribe.

Problems associated with effective record keeping not only originate from the people who use them, in terms of ambivalence and/or facilitating access, but are exacerbated by the system of record keeping itself. After prescribing a medication or other item for a patient, community nurses may need to record the information several times. This may be in their own office-based nursing or health visiting records; in the patient's notes held at the patient's home; in the parent-held child health record and in the practice or health centre based medical notes (if accessible) which may involve both written and computerised notes. This is clearly time-consuming and, when practice-based patient medical records are on a computerised system, further complications arise to confound record keeping when the system is 'down'. Access to input data may not be possible until later in the day or even the next day, resulting in an even more time-consuming backlog of information to be entered. Where nurses are not given easy or any access to patients' medical records, or where long distances need to be covered to reach practices, information sharing totally collapses as frustration over wasted journeys and time increases. Yet despite the frustrations, the pressure for health professionals to share information through records continues, directed from the first Crown Report (DoH, 1989) that stated clearly that, 'good communication between different health professionals is essential for high quality health care'.

Duplication of record keeping by health professionals may be questionable in its justification but is understandable. As individual practitioners of the primary healthcare team are not all encompassed under one legal umbrella, sharing a communal legal status (Rigby *et al*, 1998), they safeguard their own legal status by maintaining their own patient/client records. Although this may help the practitioner feel protected legally, the system prevents, 'a shared clinical perception of a patient's problems and needs' and fails to recognise the consumers' wishes for good quality, well-coordinated care (Rigby *et al*, 1998), which avoids them having to repeat their history many times to different professionals.

To solve the problem of fragmented record keeping and deficits in information sharing, there is a strong argument for the use of information technology to introduce an integrated computerised system accessible to all health professionals in the format of a single record for every patient (Clarke and Mooney, 1999; DoH, 1999). However, nurses who are currently looking for direction as to where to record information that avoids duplication and extra travelling to and from surgery will remain disappointed — the implementation process will undoubtedly be exceptionally expensive and, in keeping with what practitioners are used to in the NHS, a long time in coming. Meanwhile the practical problems of accessing records and overcoming time-consuming duplication will not only continue for some time, but have to be endured and overcome so that information is recorded in all appropriate records to ensure patient safety and provide evidence of safe practice should the nurse ever be called upon to produce it.

Implications for future prescribing

The expansion of nurse prescribing heralds a new era in nursing care in terms of placing nurses in an ever-strengthening position to extend their practice based on 'service need'. Nurses no longer need to have a health visiting or district nursing qualification to be eligible for the training to become prescribers. Instead, eligibility is based on the recognition of need within the service or services provided locally, and agreement between the nurse and employing organisation of their suitability for training to prescribe, based on professional expertise and competence.

Although any prescribing authority does and will come with adequate training and scrutiny, the prescribable substances by nurses are a far cry from 'medically insignificant' (*NPF/British National Formulary [BNF]*), and the importance of adding all prescribing events by nurses to medical notes will be even greater. The implementation guide (DoH, 2002) includes, for the first time, specifications for good practice regarding record keeping for nurses involved with prescribing. It clearly recommends that details of a nurse prescribed therapy should be entered in the nursing records (where a separate one exists) immediately, and the general patient records (GP or hospital) as soon as possible, 'preferably contemporaneously'.

Direction is clear: however insignificant the substance is considered to be, it should be recorded in all patient notes as a basis of good professional practice. Current and future decisions made by the Government surrounding the extension of nurse prescribing have been and will continue to be influenced by the level of safety and competency demonstrated by nurses involved in piloting the schemes; a significant part of which is accurate and adequate record keeping. All key stakeholders in prescribing by nurses, including the public, employers, colleagues and nurses themselves need to be totally confident that the UKCC's professional guidelines (1992a, b) provide sufficient boundaries to prevent irresponsible and unsafe prescribing by nurses, just as the British Medical Association ultimately regulates the prescribing practice of doctors (Cresswell, 1999). Recording information intelligently serves to demonstrate the nurse is working within their level of competence and is prescribing safely and appropriately. It should be remembered that the quality of record keeping reflects the standard of professional practice (UKCC, 1998).

The choice to prescribe

In view of the many arguments in support of adequate and accurate record keeping in association with nurse prescribing practice, there is no doubt that barriers to record keeping have to be overcome by the individual prescribing nurse. However, prescribing is not a compulsory part of nursing practice and is undertaken purely at the discretion of each nurse authorised to prescribe. Sometimes, when a prescribing situation appears difficult, for example, when the patient is registered at another practice and access to records is problematic or inconvenient, the decision is taken not to prescribe at all.

Luker *et al* (1997) found that in reality comparatively few practitioners were actually using their power to prescribe, with 55% of district nurses prescribing on most days, and only around 50% of health visitors prescribing, but only about once a month or less. Although there are many factors involved in why these figures are so low, anecdotally both health visitors and district nurses have reported that they have actively chosen not to prescribe. This may be associated with poor exam results, lack of confidence or competence, or problems accessing patient medical notes to record information.

Ultimately, despite the pressure to ensure record keeping is adequately maintained, nurses have the right to choose not to prescribe rather than face any threat of their professional integrity being questioned. This raises the question of whether or not the amount of money used for an indiscriminate blanket programme of nurse prescribing training was prudently spent when others may have been more than capable and, moreover, keen to train to prescribe. The new wave of nurse prescribing is welcomed insofar as it addresses this key issue taking away the restriction of nurses having to have a district nursing or health visiting qualification to access training to prescribe. This paves the way for nurses who are in an optimum position to prescribe (for example, nurse practitioners and clinical nurse specialists) to move forward to undertake the training to do so.

Conclusion

Undoubtedly, all nurses who are currently prescribing must be aware of their individual accountability and the importance of accurate and adequate record keeping. Although there are significant barriers to maintaining good record keeping, they are not an adequate defence in a court of law in the event of a case being brought against a nurse concerning prescribing practice.

With nurse prescribing now significantly expanded it is no longer information about just a mild emollient or a parasiticidal preparation to enter in a patient's notes, but the hugely extended list of significantly more potent therapies within the *Nurse Prescribers' Extended Formulary*. If deficits and inadequacies are happening now, the potential for litigation against nurse prescribers for not entering information about interventions and treatment in the appropriate place could escalate considerably. It is imperative, despite the hardships in practice, for each nurse to surmount the problems they may have in accessing patient notes, to record all prescribing information appropriately. This is not only to underpin safe practice, but to safeguard individual professional integrity. At the same time, employers of nurses need to heed the message from those choosing not to prescribe, that pushing all nurses indiscriminately through a training programme to meet their own agenda may not necessarily be prudent in terms of cost. It is more beneficial for nurses and employers to negotiate who the most willing, able and appropriate nurses are to access training to prescribe, now the Government has provided that opportunity.

Key Points

⌘ The *Nurse Prescribers' Formulary* and groups of nurses eligible to train to prescribe are set to expand.

⌘ In the interests of patient safety and to safeguard professional integrity, issues surrounding efficient record keeping in the community need to be revisited.

⌘ Prescribing nurses should ensure that they have access to all patients' records for whom they are prescribing.

References

Anderson EE (2000) Issues surrounding record keeping in district nursing practice. *Br J Community Nurs* **5**(7): 352–6

Berry L, Hurst R (1999) Nurse prescribing: the reality. In: Humphries JL, Green J, eds. *Nurse Prescribing*. Macmillan Press, London: 90–106

Clark DJ, Mooney G (1999) Primary health care records: an integrated approach. *Nurs Times* **95**(16): 48–50

Cresswell J (1998) Accountability in prescribing. *Community Nurse* **4**(2): 41–2

Cresswell J (1999) Crown Review II Report: The issues facing prescribers. *Community Nurse* **5**(7): 37–8

Department of Health (1989) *Report of the Advisory Group on Nurse Prescribing*. First Crown Report. DoH, London

Department of Health (1997) *The New NHS: Modern, Dependable*. The Stationery Office, London

Department of Health (1998) *Clinical Systems Group – Improving Clinical Communications*. DoH, Leeds

Department of Health (1999) *Review of Prescribing, Supply and Administration of Medicines – Final Report*. Crown Report. DoH, London

Department of Health (2002) *Extending Independent Nurse Prescribing within the NHS in England*. DoH, London

Dimond B (2000a) Legal issues arising in community nursing 5: nurse prescribing. *Br J Community Nurs* **5**(4): 186–9

Dimond B (2000b) Legal issues arising in community nursing 7: record keeping. *Br J Community Nurs* **5**(6): 297–9

Howse E, Bailey J (1992) Resistance to documentation: a nursing research issue. *Int J Nurs Stud* **29**(4): 371–80

Laurence DR, Bennett PN, Brown MJ (1997) *Clinical Pharmacology*. 8th edn. Churchill Livingstone, New York

Luker KA, Austin L, Willock J, Ferguson B, Smith K (1997) Nurses' and GPs' views of the Nurse Prescribers' Formulary. *Nurs Standard* **11**(22): 33–8

NHS Executive (2000) *Consultation on Proposals to Extend Nurse Prescribing*. DoH, Leeds

Rigby M, Roberts R, Williams J, Clark J, Savill A, Lervy B, Mooney G (1998) Integrated record keeping as an essential aspect of a primary care-led health service. *Br Med J* **4**(2): 41–2

Smallman S (1999) Record keeping. *Community Nurse* **4**(12): 15–6

Tingle JH (1998) Nurses must improve their record keeping skills. *Br J Nurs* **7**(5): 245

Toms EC (1992) Evaluating the quality of patient care in district nursing. *J Adv Nurs* **17**: 1489–95

United Kingdom Central Council for Nursing, Midwifery and Health Visiting (1992a) *Code of Professional Conduct for the Nurse, Midwife and Health Visitor*. UKCC, London

United Kingdom Central Council for Nursing, Midwifery and Health Visiting (1992b) *The Scope of Professional Practice*. UKCC, London

United Kingdom Central Council for Nursing, Midwifery and Health Visiting (1998) *Guidelines for Records and Record Keeping*. UKCC, London

Young A (1995) Law series 3: record keeping. *Br J Nurs* **4**(3): 179

6

Nursing management of constipation in housebound older people

Margaret Edwards, Alison Bentley

In this chapter two algorithms are suggested for use by district nurses in the management of constipation in dependent older people at home. Prescribing for this group of patients requires a complex assessment of medical and social factors as twenty-four-hour supervision is not always available and local health and social service resources may impact on the level of care that is available in terms of the provision of food and drink and the taking of medicines.

At present district nurses, together with health visitors, are legally able to prescribe those laxatives that are included in the *Nurse Prescribers' Formulary* (*NPF*) (Mehta, 1999). In the preparatory training for this prescribing role much emphasis was placed not only on the safe prescription of medicinal products but also on cost-effective prescribing (English National Board for Nursing, Midwifery and Health Visiting [ENB], 1994). Cost-effective prescribing is however a difficult task in areas such as the management of constipation where little evidence for effectiveness of treatment exists (Petticrew *et al*, 1997). Simplistic and potentially unsatisfactory conclusions can be drawn when consideration of the context of care is omitted from the cost analysis.

In this chapter, the authors have drawn on their experiences of nurse prescribing and caring for housebound older people to suggest a rational, safe approach to the management of constipation that takes into account the very real impediments and challenges faced by district nurses when attempting to deliver optimum care to the very old at home. The chapter uses the prescribing pyramid (Prescribing Nurse Bulletin, 1999) as a framework (*Figure 6.1*) for the assessment and management of care. Two algorithms are suggested to help district nurses in the decision-making process. The prescribing pyramid was found to be a useful tool for community nurses when answering examination questions during the roll-out of prescribing preparation.

The context of care

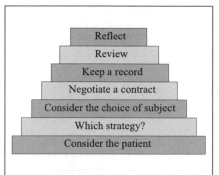

Figure 6.1: The prescribing pyramid (adapted from Prescribing Nurse Bulletin, 1999)

In the NHS there has been concern surrounding the increasing cost of laxative prescription and in particular the prescription of laxatives belonging to the more expensive group, especially co-danthramer and co-danthrusate (Petticrew *et al*, 1997). This concern is accompanied by findings that there is little information concerning the effectiveness of laxatives in older people and little evidence that the dantron laxatives represent a 'best buy for constipation' (Petticrew *et al*, 1997). The upward trend in the prescribing of laxatives preceded the roll-out of nurse prescribing so is unlikely to be attributable to the direct action of community nurses as prescribers. It is possible, however, that district nurses have influenced GP prescribing in the past by requesting particular items (Poulton and Thomas, 1999).

The systematic review of the effectiveness of laxatives in older people (Petticrew *et al*, 1997) makes an invaluable contribution to the knowledge base of the management of constipation and laxative use but, because of its particular remit, cannot throw light on the reasons why community nurses might have opted for the more expensive types of laxatives in the past or might do so in the future. The reasons for this are two-fold: there are scarcely any community studies that look specifically at those over eighty years of age living alone in the community and there is an assumption that community patients are more mobile and less dependent than hospital or nursing home patients (Petticrew *et al*, 1997).

Studies that have found constipation managed successfully with changes of diet and health promotion have tended to look at populations in institutional care, where carers have considerable control over the provision of food and drink to the subjects of the research (Beverley and Travis, 1992; Gibson *et al*, 1995). Petticrew *et al* (1997) cited Behm (1985) who found that in a nursing home sample a supplement of bran, apple sauce and prune juice resulted in reduced laxative use. In institutions, whether hospital or nursing home, care is available over the twenty-four-hour span. Interventions that are labour intensive to a degree (eg. adding bran to each meal or close supervision of drinks) are considerably easier to implement in institutions than in domiciliary settings where patients who may live alone receive intermittent visits from community nurses and/or care assistants.

The Audit Commission (1999) noted that the majority of district nursing patients were older people and that district nurses visited over half of the over-eighties. The Audit Commission also noted that more than half of those over seventy-five years old live alone. Population projections suggest that this group will continue to grow well into the twenty-first century (Royal Commission on Long Term Care for the Elderly, 1999). Conversely, the district nursing service was found to be under considerable pressure, with falling numbers and suffering from inadequate manpower planning (Audit Commission, 1999). The Commission also found that evening and night cover was not universally available. In its document, *Medicines and Older People*, the Department of Health (DoH) (2001a) makes no explicit mention of district nurses. This is curious as district nurses are independent prescribers. The failure to mention district nursing suggests that the service and the needs of its main recipients, those over eighty years of age, remain poorly understood by policy makers. The Audit Commission (1999) commented on the wealth of experience among district nurses in caring for this age group.

Surveys in both the UK and USA suggest that possibly about one-fifth of older people living in the community have symptoms of constipation (Petticrew *et al*, 1997). Although older people have been found to be receptive to health promotion (Grimley Evans, 1990) the increasing morbidity and comorbidity that is associated with advancing age (Royal Commission, 1999) may impact on whether simple, non-pharmacological approaches to the prevention and treatment of constipation are feasible or effective. Using the prescribing pyramid, consideration can be given to those factors that impinge on the management of constipation and that are unique to the setting in which district nursing is delivered.

Steps in the prescribing pyramid

Consider the patient

Patient's medical history

An overall assessment needs to be made, not only of any presenting symptoms, medical history and medication regimes but also of the patient's functional and affective status. The patient's social circumstances also need to be considered, as this will impact on the management strategy adopted in domiciliary settings. The first stage of the assessment should be to look for signs of gross pathophysiology that would require, first and foremost, medical intervention.

Defining constipation is problematic and medical and lay definitions may vary. Jones and Irving (1993) suggested that the term should be used primarily to refer to difficulty in defecation (straining) and/or infrequency, which is not secondary to some underlying cause.

Constipation can, however, be associated with a number of underlying causes, some of which require immediate medical intervention, eg. neoplastic diseases of the colon and rectum. Other causes of constipation are related to treatments for diseases, including the use of analgesics and antidepressants. In depression, there can be disturbance of neurotransmitters that can alter bio-chemical regulation, slowing down gastric and intestinal movements affecting normal eating and elimination patterns (Teahon, 1999). Diseases, such as altered mental conditions (encephalopathy, dementia, stroke) and sensory neuropathy (diabetes) may lead to constipation as they may selectively reduce conscious sensation and awareness of rectal fullness (Jorge, 1999). Taking a comprehensive health history including current medication regimes whether prescribed or purchased over the counter is therefore a necessity. Careful use of the *NPF* (Mehta *et al*, 1999) can assist in identifying those drugs that may be responsible for causing constipation in a particular patient. A detailed history of medication use may reveal long-term use of laxatives. Artificial stimulation through continual use of laxatives causes the colon to lose its natural ability to function (colonic atony). Any history of medicine taking should include noting whether the patient has particular allergies or has had an adverse reaction to particular products. Certain preparations (eg. arachis oil) have a nut basis and may cause allergic reactions.

There appears to be consensus that the range for normal bowel activity lies somewhere between three bowel motions daily to one bowel motion every three days (Drossman *et al*, 1993; Sands and Daniel, 1999). For patients it appears that symptoms such as pain and straining have greater significance than frequency (Romero *et al*, 1996). The patient's account of symptoms is pivotal in deciding the urgency and nature of nursing or other interventions. Constipation is a common presenting symptom in colorectal carcinoma (Weiss and Johnson, 1999) and the possibility of this disease being present should be in the mind of the assessor, checking in the assessment for rectal bleeding or change in bowel habit — the two most common presenting symptoms of colon and rectal cancer (Weiss and Johnson, 1999). It is important to remember that a change from three bowel motions a day to one every three days may represent a significant change for an individual patient, despite remaining within the normal limits for the population.

Abdominal pain is common in patients with colorectal cancer and pain classically attributable to neoplasms occurs secondary to partial obstruction resulting in colicky, crampy, rhythmic pain. Isolated pain in the rectum may represent rectal cancer while back pain can occur with colon cancer. Urgency, tenesmus (persistent, ineffectual spasms of the rectum) or mucus discharge may also be present (Weiss and Johnson, 1999). A thorough health assessment would note signs of advanced disease, eg. nausea, vomiting, anorexia, weight loss, lethargy, shortness of breath and chest pain, and would precipitate urgent medical referral.

Although many patients with carcinoma of the bowel have rectal bleeding, most patients with rectal bleeding do not have cancer (Weiss and Johnson, 1999). Bowel symptoms indicated above may occur with other long-standing gastrointestinal diseases, eg. inflammatory bowel disease and some common anal conditions including haemorrhoidal disease and anal fissure (Porrett and Daniel, 1999).

Patient's dietary history

Observational studies suggest that increasing fruit and fibre may be an effective approach in preventing constipation though this has not been supported by the few randomised controlled trials that have been carried out (Petticrew *et al*, 1997). These trials have not been sufficiently powered to detect real effects. There is, nonetheless, a weight of evidence in support of the hypothesis that diet has a direct influence on constipation. Petticrew *et al* (1997) pointed to studies demonstrating that dietary fibre is associated variously with increased bowel function time, faecal weight and bowel movement frequency. Studies have also demonstrated a lower incidence of constipation in vegetarians. In older adults there is some suggestion that the frequency of consumption of fruit, vegetables and bread declines significantly with age, in some cases partly due to gastro-intestinal intolerance of some of these food types or possibly as a result of chewing difficulties and denture problems in older people. Low fluid intake has been associated with constipation, slowing colonic transit time in healthy individuals or reducing stool output.

An assessment of dietary and fluid input forms an intrinsic part of any complex nursing assessment but is particularly pertinent in any assessment of the symptoms of constipation. In the community, however, the provision as well as the intake of food and drink needs to form an important part of any assessment. For patients who are not self-caring in this respect or who do not have a resident, physically and/or cognitively able carer there can be a complex array of provision, eg. social service-employed carers or contracted agency staff. Provision for housebound older people is governed by local social services department resources and there is anecdotal evidence that some departments that have exceeded their budgets have withdrawn or been unable to fund care packages for patients.

The capacity of the district nursing service to take on this type of care is limited (Audit Commission, 1999). The single assessment process and integrated provision of services which form part of *The National Service Framework for Older People* (DoH, 2001b) requirements may impact positively here but there is no guarantee that joint commissioning will make up for the current shortfall in manpower in both agencies.

Mobility

The patient's level of mobility may be linked to his/her symptoms of constipation. It has been hypothesised that levels of activity may enhance high amplitude motor contractions in the colon causing contraction waves propelling faeces onwards. These typically occur on walking and following meals (Jorge, 1999). Lack of mobility may slow colonic transit time.

Linked to problems of mobility is the need to assess the physical environment. Declining mobility may make the toilet either inaccessible or difficult to reach. Immobile patients at home may be dependent on visiting carers for toileting, disrupting the individual's natural elimination patterns.

Acute vs chronic

It is important in the assessment process to distinguish between acute constipation for which there is an explanation, eg. recent change of routine, change of diet, episode of febrile illness or hospitalisation, and that which is of a chronic nature suggesting the need for further investigation. The Rome diagnostic criteria (Thompson *et al*, 1992) may be a useful tool. According to the Rome criteria, a diagnosis of constipation requires two or more of the following symptoms to be present for at least three months:

- straining at defecation for at least a quarter of the time
- lumpy and/or hard stools for at least a quarter of the time
- a sensation of incomplete evacuation for at least a quarter of the time
- two or fewer bowel movements per week.

Strategies and choice of product

Having excluded the need for urgent medical intervention or review, the choice of strategy will be guided by the history. Immediate presenting symptoms need to be dealt with first. Where the patient complains of feeling constipated and is experiencing discomfort a rectal examination is indicated. The law (Medicinal Products: Prescription by Nurses etc Act, 1992) permits district nurses, as independent prescribers, to prescribe items from a limited formulary. Implicit in this is the need to carry out relevant diagnostic procedures. Over the last few years there has been mounting confusion around the subject of rectal examination. Royal College of Nursing guidelines (Addison *et al*, 1995) recommend that nurses undertaking digital examination are 'appropriately trained'. In some clinical areas it has come to be the rule that no-one may undertake a rectal examination without specialist training. This blanket prohibition may cause unacceptable delay in patients receiving a necessary diagnostic procedure.

Confusion arises because checking for a loaded rectum has come to be seen in the same light as carrying out a full rectal examination such as that by nurse specialists (Addison, 1999) to exclude rectal pathology. One fear is that nurses may damage the rectum while performing a check. In preparing this chapter the authors undertook a search of Medline and CINAHL databases (1966–2000) but were unable to uncover any published evidence of perforation of the rectum by district nurses (or indeed by any other nurse) managing constipation. Personal communication with peers and colorectal nurse specialists similarly failed to uncover any known cases. If these exist they do not do so in any number to warrant publication of the data. It may be assumed that before nurse prescribing and the administration of enemas or suppositories by nurses, rectal examinations in the community were always carried out by GPs. GPs and district nurses know otherwise. Any cases of nurse-induced perforation need to be balanced against the number of rectal examinations that have been carried out by nurses without any adverse event.

District nurses need to be reassured by the singular lack of evidence that their training is inadequate for the purpose of detecting a loaded rectum and also by the fact that perforation of the rectum even by rigid sigmoidoscope is rare (Sands and Daniel, 1999). Indeed the rectum is often recommended as a site for biopsy because it is surrounded by a number of muscular structures. Nurse prescribing has the potential to bring immediate relief to patients. Illogical retreat to rule-bound practice runs counter to the scope of professional practice and nurse prescribing and could be considered as a contravention of the code of professional practice where the nurse must weigh up issues not only of not doing harm but also the obligation to do good.

The choice of product will depend on the consistency of the stool found on examination (*Figures 6.2* and *6.3*). It is important to remember that it is anatomically impossible to conclude that the rectum is empty through simple digital examination. The length of the rectum (approximately 15cm) is beyond the reach of the longest index fingers. The patient's history will therefore guide the need to give a suppository or enema.

Where the patient is passing faeces but the stool is hard and difficult to pass, involving straining and discomfort, the strategy will depend on:

❖ Whether the patient is amenable to changing his/her fluid and dietary intake and whether a stepped approach, eg. increasing fluid and dietary fibre before recourse to laxatives (Petticrew *et al*, 1997) may be used. Barrett (1992) suggested that bulking agents in older people may increase the risk of faecal incontinence. Faecal impaction with overflow should always be considered when an older patient presents with diarrhoea (Stuchfield and Eccersley, 1999).

❖ Will the patient be willing or able to drink sufficient fluids to accompany the prescription of a bulk-forming laxative? Eight to ten cups of fluid (excluding tea or coffee) is a recommended daily intake (Weiss and Johnson, 1999).

❖ Is close supervision of fluid intake possible throughout a twenty-four-hour period?

❖ Do the patient's other medical conditions prohibit an increase in fluid intake, eg. degree of heart failure or renal failure?

❖ Does a lack of mobility prevent the prescription of a bulk-forming laxative?

Where oral laxatives are indicated consideration should be given as to how and when these should be taken, eg. can the patient self-medicate or is help or supervision needed?

If local resources do not allow for supervision of the medication that is to be taken several times a day or at night it may be more cost-effective to prescribe a relatively expensive product such as compound macrogol oral powder, which can be taken once a day; the authors have recently learned of a case where an older person was brought to a walk-in centre in the evening requiring treatment for constipation and had to be referred to the local accident and emergency department. Multicompartment compliance aids (DoH, 2001a) can be of use but still present difficulties for patients with reduced cognitive function, poor manual dexterity or those who need to take medicines in liquid form.

Consideration needs to be given to the time taken by the preparation to act as this can vary between preparations. Senna may act within eight hours while lactulose may take up to seventy-two hours to work (Mehta, 1999). Choosing a senna/lactulose combination means that taken together they will act at different times. It is perhaps easy to see why prescribing a more expensive preparation such as co-danthramer or macrogol which has a more predictable and shorter working time may be seen as more suitable and effective for the community patient. Medicines in the dantron group are licensed only for use with the terminally ill and for older people where straining is contraindicated (ie. those with cardiac failure or coronary thrombosis). Macrogol may be prescribed for constipation. It may be prescribed for faecal impaction but only after medical review (Mehta, 1999). The addition of linseed to food is sometimes recommended and gentle massage of the abdomen over the colon in the direction of peristalsis may be helpful, particularly where there is diverticular disease (Taylor, 1999).

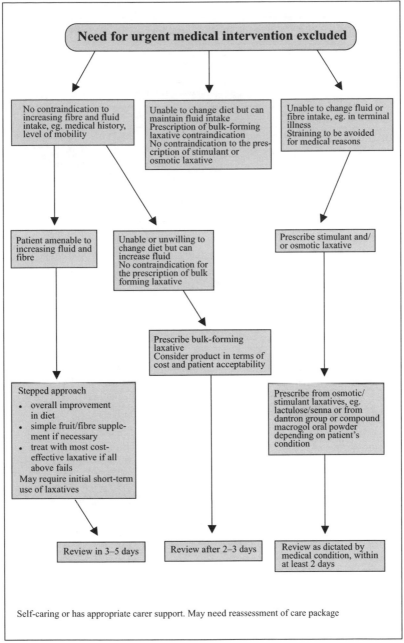

Figure 6.2: Symptom management algorithm for use with patients passing infrequent hard stools

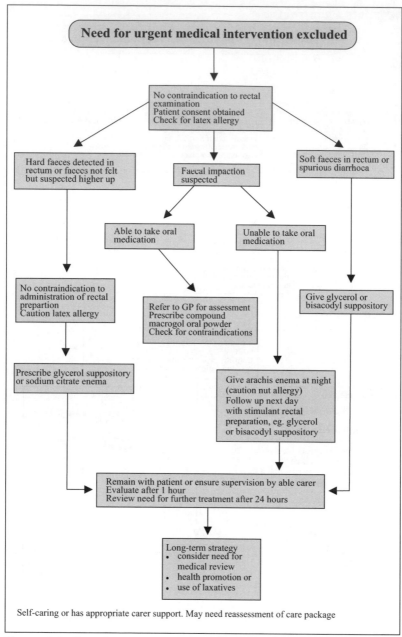

Figure 6.3: Symptom management algorithm for use with patients complaining of acute discomfort and a history of not passing motions for more than three days

Negotiate a contract

In implementing a strategy the consent and agreement of the patient is paramount. A patient may be unable to give informed consent, eg. in the case of a patient with dementia who is perhaps experiencing faecal impaction with spurious diarrhoea. Long-term care may involve the use of regular enemas to keep the rectum free of faeces (Stuchfield and Eccersley, 1999). Communication with carers and the patient's GP is important here but in the absence of indication that informed consent is possible the district nurse would be best served to apply the principles of ethical decision making in invoking the need to do good and prevent harm.

The patient needs to know what is expected of him/her in carrying out the treatment plan and when the nurse intends to reassess the situation. Patients should be alerted to any known side-effects and should have access to the product information sheets that accompany dispensed medicines. The side-effects of the group of medicines can be alarming if the patient or carer has not been alerted to the fact that tears or urine may be stained red. On occasions, judgement is required in deciding how much information should be imparted. In law the nurse will be expected to have behaved in a similar vein to the 'prudent doctor' (*Sidaway* v. *Board of Governors of Bethlem Royal Hospital*, [1985]). Informal carers and other statutory carers, eg. social service care assistants, may be expected to contribute to the care plan. They need to be appraised of instructions for encouraging a high-fibre diet and the need to take sufficient fluids.

Record keeping

Not only do patients and carers need to be appraised of treatments, but other professionals, including GPs, need to have relevant information to inform their own treatments and to avoid poly-pharmacy and adverse events from drug interactions.

Information needs to be recorded in the patient's nursing notes and the patient's medical records. Since the roll-out of nurse prescribing the recording of prescriptions and advice given has exercised the ingenuity of managers and district nurses alike. Duplicate forms have been used but anecdotal evidence suggests that they are not popular in those GP practices that operate on a paper-free basis. Forms can simply be placed in the notes adding to the bulk but not the quality of the recording. The need to develop good systems for communicating prescribing advice is urgent, particularly when other nurses and health professionals are able to become prescribers.

Review and reflect

The review of nursing management of constipation will be directly related to the diagnosis and the strategy undertaken. Lifestyle changes will take time to effect bowel habit changes. Likewise, results in stool consistency or ease of passage of stools may not be apparent for three days or more when certain groups of laxatives are used. *Figures 6.2* and *6.3* suggest review times related to health promotion and medicinal interventions. The interplay between a complex clinical situation where there may be many different causes of presenting symptoms of constipation as well as difficult social circumstances, calls for careful review of prescribing and treatment decisions. With little research available to help the district nurse prevent and treat constipation in dependent older people at home, practice reviews that can be shared through clinical supervision may help to guide practice and lay the basis for research in this area.

Conclusion

In this chapter the authors have tried to explore the management of constipation in older people at home from a district nursing perspective. Two algorithms for safe management are suggested in *Figures 6.2* and *6.3*. In the community, among dependent older people at home, the use of more expensive preparations may be the most cost-effective option, otherwise the cost may be borne by other parts of the NHS such as accident and emergency departments.

There are relatively few studies of interventions among older people living in the community. There are even less dealing with the very old living at home. Petticrew *et al* (1997) rightly called for studies that include more detailed subgroup analysis which they claim would permit different treatments to be targeted at the appropriate patient group. The standards laid out in the medicine-related aspects of *The National Service Framework for Older People* (DoH, 2001b) are useful in trying to ensure that a high quality service is available to this set of patients, but they fall short of acknowledging that preventing and managing constipation in dependent older people at home is a labour-intensive business, where prescribing must sometimes be tailored to the patient's social circumstances and to the availability of local health and social care resources.

Key Points

⌘ Managing constipation in the housebound elderly requires a complex assessment of medical and social factors.

⌘ Prescribing decisions by district nurses have to be evaluated in relation to the context of care.

⌘ There is no evidence that district nurses lack the expertise to carry out rectal examinations to check for constipation.

⌘ Algorithms may be useful in guiding prescribing decisions.

References

Addison R (1999) Digital rectal examination 2. *Nurs Times* **95**(41): Suppl 1–2

Addison R, Duffin H, Miles B *et al* (1995) *Rectal Examination and Removal of Faeces: The Role of the Nurse.* Royal College of Nursing, London

Audit Commission (1999) *First Assessment: A Review of District Nursing Services in England and Wales.* Audit Commission, London

Barrett JA (1992) Colorectal disorders in elderly people. *Br Med J* **305**: 764–6

Behm RA (1985) A special recipe to banish constipation. *Geriatric Nurs* **6**: 216–7

Beverley L, Travis I (1992) Constipation: proposed natural laxative mixtures. *J Gerontol Nurs* **18**(10): 5–12

Department of Health (2001a) *Medicines and Older People. Implementing Medicines-related Aspects of the NSF for Older People.* The Stationery Office, London

Department of Health (2001b) *The National Service Framework for Older People.* The Stationery Office, London

Drossman DA, Li Z, Andruzzi E *et al* (1993) US householder survey of functional gastrointestinal disorders. Prevalence, sociodemography and health impact. *Dig Dis Sci* **38**: 1569–80

English National Board (1994) *Nurse Prescribing Open Learning Pack.* ENB, London

Gibson CJ, Opalka PC, Moore CA, Brady RS, Mion LC (1995) Effectiveness of bran supplement on the bowel management of elderly rehabilitation patients. *J Gerontol Nurs* **21**(10): 21–30

Grimley Evans J (1990) Quality of life assessments in older people. In: Hopkins A, ed. *Measures of the Quality of Life and the Use to Which Such Measures May be Put.* Royal College of Physicians Publications, London: 107–17

Jones DJ, Irving MH (1993) *ABC of Colorectal Diseases.* BMJ Publishing Group, London

Jorge JMN (1999) Anatomy and physiology of the colon, rectum and anus. In: Porrett T, Daniel N, eds. *Essential Coloproctology for Nurses.* Whurr Publishers, London: 21–51

Mehta D, ed (1999) *Nurse Prescribers' Formulary 1999–2001.* British Medical Association/Royal Pharmaceutical Society of Great Britain, London

Petticrew M, Watt I, Sheldon T (1997) Systematic review of the effectiveness of laxatives in the elderly. *Health Technology Assessment* **1**(13): i–iv, 1–52

Porrett T, Daniel N, eds (1999) *Essential Coloproctology for Nurses.* Whurr Publishers, London

Poulton B, Thomas S (1999) The nursing cost of constipation. *Primary Health Care* November: 1–5

Prescribing Nurse Bulletin (1999) Signposts for prescribing nurses: general principles of good prescribing. 1(1) National Prescribing Centre, Liverpool

Romero Y, Evans JM, Fleming KC, Philips SF (1996) Constipation and fecal incontinence in the elderly population. *Mayo Clin Proc* **71**: 81–92

Royal Commission on Long Term Care for the Elderly (1999) Chairman Sir Stuart Sutherland *With Respect to Old Age, Long Term Care — Rights and Responsibilities*. Cm 4192-1. The Stationery Office, London

Sands LR, Daniel N (1999) Investigation and examination of a patient with colorectal problems. In: Porrett T, Daniel N, eds. *Essential Coloproctology for Nurses*. Whurr Publishers, London: 52–75

Schoetz DJ (1993) Uncomplicated diverticulitis: indications for surgery and surgical management. *Surg Clin North Am* **73**(5): 965–74

Sidaway v. *Board of Governors of Bethlem Royal Hospital* [1985] AC 871

Stuchfield B, Eccersley AJP (1999) The modern management of faecal incontinence. In: Porrett T, Daniel N, eds. *Essential Coloproctology for Nurses*. Whurr Publishers, London: 292–317

Taylor P (1999) Irritable bowel syndrome. In: Porrett T, Daniel N, eds. *Essential Coloproctology for Nurses*. Whurr Publishers, London: 222–55

Teahon E (1999) Constipation. In: Porrett T, Daniel N, eds. *Essential Coloproctology for Nurses*. Whurr Publishers, London: 206–21

Thompson WG, Creed F, Drossman DA, Heaton KW (1992) Functional bowel disease and functional abdominal pain. *Gastroenterol Int* **5**(2): 75–91

Weiss EG, Johnson TE (1999) Colorectal cancer. In: Porrett T, Daniel N, eds. *Essential Coloproctology for Nurses*. Whurr Publishers, London: 97–118

7

Assess, negotiate, treat: community prescribing for chronic wounds

Jenny Bentley

The cost of prescribing wound-care products in general practice in 1999 exceeded £95 million (Department of Health [DoH], 1999a). However, there is a lack of randomised controlled trials to assess the effectiveness of wound-care products (National Prescribing Centre, 1999a) and there is evidence that non-effective treatments are being prescribed (DoH, 1999a). Use of the prescribing pyramid, as taught during nurse prescribing courses, may help community nurses justify their decisions and assess their wound-care practices. Wounds commonly encountered in the community include pressure sores, leg ulcers, fungating wounds and cavity wounds. The ideal choice of product is one that allows moist wound healing, is cost effective, clinically effective and acceptable to the patient.

Dressing wounds is a major feature of community nursing work. One of the reasons for implementing nurse prescribing was the recognition that time was being wasted in nurses requesting prescriptions for dressings (Department of Health, 1986).

With newly qualified prescribers in the community, the need for ongoing support was identified, and one of the first Prescribing Nurse Bulletins (National Prescribing Centre, 1999a), commissioned by the NHS Executive, provided guidance on modern wound-management dressings. In this bulletin, the need for wound assessment was emphasised. While ongoing education for nurses was one stimulus for these guidelines, another possible incentive was cost. In 1999, the cost of wound-care products prescribed in general practice in England was estimated to exceed £95 million (DoH, 1999a). Since wound-care products are the most frequently prescribed items by district nursing prescribers (Luker *et al*, 1997), careful assessment of the effectiveness of the management of the wound should be part of every nurse prescriber's practice.

Using the nurse prescribing pyramid (*Figure 7.1*), often emphasised during nurse prescribing training, this chapter will address the management of chronic wounds, which community nurses may encounter in their daily practice in relation to the *Nurse Prescribers' Formulary* (*NPF*) (Mehta, 1999). The chapter will also examine the implications for independent prescribers, as defined by the second Crown Report (DoH, 1999b).

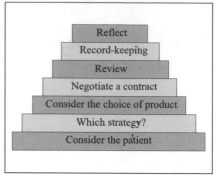

Figure 7.1: The nurse prescribing pyramid (National Prescribing Centre, 1999b)

Consider the patient

The nursing assessment should not focus exclusively on the wound, but must take a holistic approach. The effects of the wound on body image, psychological health and social function are important elements in an assessment, and acknowledgement of these issues may increase patient concordance and foster a partnership relationship with the patient. Recognition of the developmental dimensions of wound healing, such as the increased healing time associated with the ageing process, may enable more realistic goals, such as estimated healing times, to be set. Existing medical conditions, eg. diabetes mellitus and anaemia, will influence wound healing, and monitoring and treatment of underlying pathology requires a team approach. Patients with diabetes are particularly vulnerable to complications and infection in wounds, and should have their wounds checked more frequently.

Chronic wounds, by definition, are not quick to heal. Many factors may be responsible for delayed wound healing (*Table 7.1*). Chronic wounds commonly encountered in the community are:

- pressure ulcers
- leg ulcers
- fungating wounds
- cavity wounds: sinuses and fistulae.

Table 7.1: Factors that delay wound healing

Factor	Example
Adverse conditions at the wound site	Presence of foreign or dead material
Pathophysiological factors	Malnutrition, vascular disease
Adverse effect of other therapies	Prolonged steroids, chemotherapy
Inappropriate wound management	Inappropriate dressings
Increasing age	Decreased epidermal-cell replacement

Source: Morison *et al*, 1997

Pressure ulcers

Pressure ulcers have been defined as a local area of damage to the skin and underlying tissue, usually over bony prominences, caused by pressure, shear or friction; the damage persists after the removal of pressure (NHS Centre for Research and Dissemination [NHSCRD], 1995). Pressure relief to prevent further damage in a susceptible patient must be included in the plan of care, as should an adequate nutritional intake. When the wound itself is examined, the extent of the damage should be assessed. A classification tool may be useful. The Stirling Index (Reid and Morison, 1994) is an attempt to reach standardisation in the classification of pressure sores; standardisation is essential to the accurate measurement of prevalence and incidence (Phillips, 1997) as part of the clinical governance agenda.

Leg ulcers

A leg ulcer is a non-healing breakdown of epidermal and dermal tissue, below the knee on the leg or foot, due to any cause (Moffatt and Harper, 1997). Determination of the aetiology of the wound, by a comprehensive assessment that includes Doppler ultrasound, is essential for appropriate and safe management of the ulcer, as well as for the setting of realistic goals for healing. Common causes of ulceration include venous disease, arterial disease and diabetes mellitus. Compression therapy is the mainstay for management of venous disease, but is contraindicated in arterial disease, which increases the need for accurate assessment.

Fungating wounds

Ulceration and proliferation are features of fungating wounds, and are caused by the invasion of malignant cells through the skin; sinus and fistula formation may complicate these wounds (Grocott, 1995). Hypoxia, tissue necrosis, odour and infection may all be unpleasant aspects of these wounds. The focus for wound management is palliative (Morison *et al*, 1997). Attention to the patient's psychological health is an important part of the holistic assessment.

Cavity wounds

Sinuses are blind-ended tracts lined with epithelium and granulation tissue; cutaneous fistulae are abnormal tracts between two epithelial surfaces that connect a viscus to the skin (Morison *et al*, 1997). Examples of sinuses commonly encountered in the community are pilonidal sinuses and post-operative sinuses. An example is a fistula connecting the gastrointestinal tract to the skin, where there are nutritional implications for the patient.

Wound assessment

After the cause, aetiology and group of the wound have been established, other factors to be alert to are:

- tissue type: necrotic, sloughy, granulating, epithelialising
- exudate: heavy, moderate, light
- size and dimensions
- signs of clinical infection: increased exudate, erythema, increased pain, odour
- state of surrounding skin (National Prescribing Centre, 1999a).

Many local trusts have their own wound-assessment chart which, together with wound mapping or photography, facilitates ongoing monitoring of the wound.

Assessment findings form the basis of rational decision making (Morison *et al*, 1997), and the importance of an accurate, comprehensive, holistic assessment cannot be overstated for the effective management of care.

Which strategy?

The plan of care for every type of chronic wound mentioned in this chapter will involve some form of dressing. Education and involvement of patients should be included in the plan. For the purpose of providing holistic care, it may be in the patient's best interests to involve other members of the primary care team. The general practitioner, for example, will need to be involved if infection is suspected, or if an underlying condition (eg. anaemia) needs to be corrected. Complex wounds may require the expertise of a colleague with specialist knowledge. Patients with reduced mobility and limited joint movement may benefit from a referral to the physiotherapist. Nutritional deficits may warrant referral to a dietitian, or social services may need to be involved for assistance with meal preparation. If the wound is in a difficult area, eg. the sacrum, moving and handling aids may be needed.

Choice of product

There is currently no single product that fulfils all the requirements of an ideal wound dressing (*Box 7.1*) although the principles in *Box 7.1* are important in the promotion of moist wound healing. There is also a lack of randomised controlled trials that assess the effectiveness of wound-care products (National Prescribing Centre, 1999a).

Box 7.1: Characteristics of the ideal wound dressing

The ideal wound dressing should:

❖ Maintain high humidity at wound/dressing interface but avoid maceration
❖ Allow gaseous exchange
❖ Provide thermal insulation and the optimal temperature for wound healing
❖ Be free of particles and safe (non-toxic; non-sensitising)
❖ Be impermeable to micro-organisms
❖ Be non-adherent and reduce the need for frequent redressing
❖ Be cost-effective

Source: Morgan, 2000

The remaining charts and information in this chapter about products may help community nurses make an informed choice from the *NPF*. Examples and main features of some *NPF* products are given in *Table 7.2*. I will give a brief outline of specific requirements of the chronic wounds under discussion.

Pressure ulcers

The assessment of the wound — including its appearance, the state of the surrounding skin, exudate and site — will decide the type of dressing required for pressure ulcers. *Table 7.3* shows suitable products for different wound types. Although enzymes (streptokinase-streptodornase products) are in the *NPF* and are included as a treatment for necrotic wounds, they are not particularly cost-effective; they require daily renewal and reconstitution, which adds to the time spent changing the dressing.

The site of the wound may indicate the need for a dressing with a water-repellent backing. A bordered hydrocolloid, for example, might be the product of choice for a pressure ulcer on the sacrum of an incontinent patient. Heels are difficult areas to dress; although shaped dressings are available, they tend to be more costly than normal dressings. The cutting and overlapping of strips of dressings, such as foams and hydrocolloids, may allow this difficulty to be overcome.

Leg ulcers

Patients with venous leg ulcers are treated with compression therapy, provided that arterial disease has been excluded. In a multilayer system, the primary wound layer is commonly a non-adherent dressing. Although other products can be used successfully, consideration should be given to the function of the dressing in handling moisture content, which may be impaired by bandages. As with other wounds, the state of the surrounding skin must be taken into account. Sensitive or inflamed skin may be worsened by adhesives in dressings, or by components of some moisturisers, so bland dressings and non-allergenic moisturisers are the preferred treatment option in such cases. If the compression method in use is short-stretch bandaging or elastic hosiery, dressings with an adhesive border may be more appropriate.

Table 7.2: Examples and main features of NPF products

Product type	Examples currently in NPF	Characteristics	Comments
Hydrocolloids	Comfeel® (Coloplast, Peterborough) Granuflex® (ConvaTec, Uxbridge) Tegasorb® (3M, Bracknell)	Promote autolytic debridement Promote angiogenesis Require changing every 3–6 days	Require margin of 2cm from wound edge Use with caution in infected wounds
Hydrogels	Intrasite® (Smith & Nephew, Hull) Nu-Gel® (Johnson & Johnson, Maidenhead) Purilon® Gel (Coloplast)	Rehydrate Promote autolysis Effective for 1–3 days	Avoid in heavily exuding and/or infected wounds
Alginates	Algisite®M (Smith & Nephew) Kaltogel® (Convatec) Sorbsan® (Maersk, Worcester)	Highly absorbent Form gel with exudate Can be irrigated from wound	Avoid in lightly exuding or dry wounds Avoid over-packing in wound
Foams	Allevyn® (Smith & Nephew) Lyofoam Extra® (SSL, Cheshire) Tielle® (3M)	Provide thermal insulation Absorbent Require changing every 3–7 days	Avoid on dry wounds Substantial variation in price
Films	Cutifilm® (Beiersdorf, Milton Keynes) Opsite® Flexigrid (Smith & Nephew) Tegaderm® (3M)	Comfortable Secondary dressings for gels Enable observation	May cause maceration Avoid unless exudate is light
Low adherent (knitted viscose)	N-A Ultra® (Johnson & Johnson) Tricotex® (Smith & Nephew)	Non-allergenic	
Carbonated dressings	Actisorb Silver 220® (Johnson & Johnson)	Absorb odour Bactericidal	Avoid in lightly exuding wounds
Iodine dressings	Inadine® (Johnson & Johnson) Iodoflex® (Smith & Nephew) Iodosorb® (Smith & Nephew)	Antimicrobial	Avoid in iodine sensitivity, thyroid disorders, pregnancy

Table 7.3: Choice of wound-care products for chronic wounds (primary wound layer)

Exuding wound type	Heavy exudate	Medium exudate	Light exudate
Necrotic	Alginates* Foams	Hydrocolloids Hydrogels* Alginates*	Hydrocolloids Hydrogels*
Sloughy	Alginates* Foams	Hydrocolloids Hydrogels* Alginates*	Hydrocolloids Hydrogels*
Granulating	Alginates* Foams	Hydrocolloids Foams	Hydrocolloids Films Non-adherent*
Epithelialising	Alginates* Foams	Foams Films	Films Non-adherent*

*Requires secondary dressing: adds to dressing cost

Fungating wounds

The main principles of wound management in these wounds are to control bleeding, exudate and odour (Morgan, 2000), rather than to promote healing. Carbonated dressings may be useful in masking odour, but there is currently a limited choice of such products in the *NPF*. Iodine products may be useful in controlling infection, but their use should be of short duration if the wound is large, since iodine may be systemically absorbed. However, the patient may find the colour and presentation of Iodosorb® and Iodoflex® (Smith & Nephew, Hull) unacceptable. Other factors for patients with these wounds are the need to avoid bulky dressings and the effect of the wound on body image. A combination of products will probably be required, such as carbon dressings, plus an alginate, plus a foam. Redressing is often required on a daily basis.

Cavity wounds

Products specifically intended for cavity wounds are a recent addition in the *Drug Tariff* (DoH, 2001). Hydrogels and alginate rope are the preferred products to fill the cavity, and are normally easy to remove by irrigation. Their use enables a patient with a pilonidal sinus to have a shower at a pre-arranged time, so that the community nurse is presented with a clean, irrigated wound ready to dress, and the patient is able to maintain adequate personal hygiene. Alginates should not be packed too tightly, since undue pressure can be exerted, causing pain to the patient. Foams are convenient as secondary dressings.

Fistulae may be discharging enzyme-rich contents that will affect skin condition. The management of fistulae need not be limited to wound-care products — an appropriate stoma bag will protect the skin and contain the odour.

Negotiate a contract

The involvement of patients in the decisions taken regarding their care is a fundamental requirement for adherence, since wound healing may be adversely affected by practices based on the patient's own beliefs (Hallett *et al*, 2000). In my own clinical experience, patients may hold the opinion that, 'leaving wounds open to the air helps them heal'. Such beliefs require sensitive handling and an open discussion about the suitability of specific strategies.

An explanation in lay terms of how the wound-care product works, and how often it should be replaced, should be included in a patient's education. Not acknowledging the patient's experience, ignoring reported dressing discomfort, and failing to act on this information, may influence non-adherence (Papadopoulos and Jukes, 1999). Attention given to the cause of the wound, as well as to the associated symptoms, could be an important element in patient education.

As part of the promotion of a patient's involvement in his/her care, the patient's viewpoint should be sought and, if appropriate, their active involvement too — such as doing their own dressings to fit in with their lifestyle, provided that the community nurse has taught them what to do and frequently monitors the progress of the wound. Owing to the usual sites of pressure sores, and the debility of patients with such wounds, involvement may not be a fitting strategy for the management of pressure sores. However, the relief of pressure remains a prime topic for the education of patients.

Review

In terms of prescribing, no more than six repeat prescriptions should be given without reviewing the patient (National Prescribing Centre, 1999b). Most wounds encountered in the community will need redressing at least once a week, thus giving regular opportunities for assessment of the wound's progress. Professional judgement and trust policies will dictate the minimal time lapse before reassessment — which may also include assessment of risk and of the efficacy of preventive strategies, which in turn will inform quality of care measurements as part of clinical governance.

The review should identify the cost and clinical effectiveness of the nursing intervention and choice of product, and also its acceptability to the patient.

Wound-mapping and photography may assist in the assessment of clinical effectiveness. Certain products, eg. OpSite® Flexigrid (Smith & Nephew), include measuring tools in the packaging.

Cost-effectiveness will be measured by the prescribing analysis and cost (PACT) data, although community nurses have ready access to current costs of products via the latest editions of the *Drug Tariff* (DoH, 2001) and *British National Formulary* (*BNF*) (Mehta, 2001).

The possibility of adverse drug reaction should not be forgotten with wound-care products, especially those that are iodine-based (Mehta, 1999) and any self-medication in the form of skin creams. At present, only a physician can report an adverse reaction to the Committee on Safety of Medicines through the yellow-card scheme. This regulation highlights the need for communication, one of the factors involved in prescribing in a team context. It may also be prudent to discuss the use and effectiveness of expensive wound-care products with the GP.

Record keeping

Accurate and timely record keeping, which is an integral part of nursing practice, promotes safety and continuity of care; the quality of record keeping is a reflection of the standard of a nurse's professional practice (UKCC, 1998). In wound-care prescribing, there is an additional requirement to document on the patient's medical notes the prescriptions that have been issued. When these are computerised, certain computer programmes, such as Egton Medical Information Systems (EMIS), allow monitoring of usage and cost.

Documentation of the progress of the wound makes it possible to assess the quality of the care delivered, and will assist in clinical audit. Audit is part of the clinical governance agenda and is also a component of risk management, of which the ultimate aim is the promotion of quality (UKCC, 1998). Measuring tools help in the assessment of wound progress and the effectiveness of interventions.

Reflect

Reviewing and reflecting on prescribing decisions assists nurses in improving their practice (National Prescribing Centre, 1999a), particularly in the absence of firm evidence of the comparative effectiveness of products (National Prescribing Centre, 1999b). The choice of dressing product should be the most effective in terms of cost and patient outcome; the cheapest is not always the most cost-effective, especially if more frequent dressings are needed, which increases both product costs and nursing time.

Being accountable involves being answerable to decisions taken, and the onus is firmly on the nurse prescriber to account for his/her actions. Evidence suggests that products that do not fulfil the criteria for the ideal wound dressing (*Box 7.1*), such as gauze and plastic-backed absorbent pads, are still widely prescribed (DoH, 1999a). The use of such products should be questioned. Part of the difficulty may be that such products are still included in the *Drug Tariff* (DoH, 2001) while other products, which conform more closely to the characteristics of the ideal wound dressing (*Box 7.1*) received slow acceptance for inclusion (Heenan, 1997); recent examples are products for malodorous and cavity wounds.

The cost to the patient, not only regarding quality of life but also in financial terms, should be taken into account — especially if that patient is paying for prescriptions. Over-the-counter treatments are rarely a viable alternative for modern, effective, wound-care products, which tend to be expensive.

Finally, post-registration education and practice (PREP) requirements indicate that nurses should keep up-to-date in developments in practice (UKCC, 2001) so that they can deliver the best possible care for patients.

Key Points

⌘ Holistic assessment of patients is the basis on which decisions of wound-care management should be made.

⌘ Chronic wound care requires a multidisciplinary approach.

⌘ The choice of product should promote moist wound healing and take into account the stage of healing, the amount of exudate and the condition of the surrounding skin.

⌘ Use of the prescribing pyramid can help nurses to prescribe safely and effectively.

⌘ Safe and effective prescribing is part of the clinical governance agenda.

References

Department of Health (1986) *Neighbourhood Nursing: A Focus for Care*. DoH, London

Department of Health (1999a) Prescription cost analysis: England 1999. http://www.doh.gov.uk/stats/pca99.htm (accessed 28.2.01)

Department of Health (1999b) *Review of Prescribing, Supply and Administration of Medicines (Crown Report)*. DoH, London

Department of Health (2001) *Drug Tariff*. March. The Stationery Office, London

Grocott P (1995) The palliative management of fungating malignant wounds. *J Wound Care* 4(5): 240–42

Hallett CE, Austin L, Caress A, Luker KA (2000) Community nurses' perceptions of patient 'compliance' in wound care: a discourse analysis. *J Adv Nurs* 32(1): 115–23

Heenan A (1997) *Dressing on the Drug Tariff*. Rev. 4.0. http://www.smtl.co.uk/World-Wide-Wounds/1997/july/Heenan/Tariff.html

Luker K, Austin L, Willcock J, Ferguson B, Smith K (1997) Nurses and GPs' views of the Nurse Prescribers' Formulary. *Nurs Standard* 11(22): 33–8

Mehta DK, ed (1999) *Nurse Prescribers' Formulary 1999–2001*. British Medical Association/Royal Pharmaceutical Society of Great Britain, London

Mehta, DK, ed (2001) *British National Formulary*. British Medical Association/Royal Pharmaceutical Society of Great Britain, London

Moffatt C, Harper P (1997) *Leg Ulcers*. Churchill Livingstone, Edinburgh

Morgan D (2000) *Formulary of Wound Management Products*. 8th edn. Uromed Communications, Haslemere

Morison M, Moffatt C, Bridel-Nixon J, Bale S (1997) *Nursing Management of Chronic Wounds*. 2nd edn. Mosby, London

National Prescribing Centre (1999a) Modern wound management dressings. *Prescrib Nurse Bull* 1(2): 5–8

National Prescribing Centre (1999b) *Principles of good prescribing*. Prescribing Nurse Factsheet 3

NHS Centre for Research and Dissemination (1995) The prevention and treatment of pressure sores. *Effective Health Care Bulletin* 2(1)

Papadopoulos A, Jukes R (1999) Motivation and compliance in wound management. *J Wound Care* 8(9): 467–9

Phillips J (1997) *Pressure Sores*. Churchill Livingstone, Edinburgh

Reid J, Morison M (1994) Towards a consensus: classification of pressure sores. *J Wound Care* 3(3): 157–60

United Kingdom Central Council for Nursing, Midwifery and Health Visiting (1998) *Standards for Records and Record Keeping*. UKCC, London

United Kingdom Central Council for Nursing, Midwifery and Health Visiting (2001) *The PREP Handbook*. UKCC, London

8

Compression hosiery in venous insufficiency: a natural nurse-led field

Dianne Bowskill

The use of compression hosiery for the treatment and prevention of venous ulceration caused by venous insufficiency is commonplace in community practice. In recent years the role of the nurse in the management of these patients has grown supported by increasing levels of knowledge, nurse specialists and the implementation of nurse prescribing. The full list of compression hosiery items available on NHS prescription are included in the list of nurse prescribing items in the Nurse Prescribers' Formulary and the Drug Tariff. Central to a successful treatment outcome is the patient assessment. This forms the base for a partnership approach to care upon which product choices and advice can be tailored to meet the individual needs of that patient. An understanding of venous physiology, limb measurement skills and hosiery care place the nurse in an ideal position to lead in this area of nursing practice.

Compression hosiery garments are used in the prevention and treatment of venous hypertension and are prescribed to help prevent recurrent ulceration or as an alternative to compression bandaging. Hosiery garments are available as below-knee socks, thigh-length stockings and tights. Compression hosiery garments are available in the community as prescription items listed in the *Drug Tariff* (part 1XA) — tights are not included in the list and therefore not available on prescription.

Patients who require a prescription for hosiery have in the past been referred to the GP. The prescription written by the GP would give details of the hosiery classification and the supply quantity but would generally leave limb measurement and product choice to the pharmacist (Mishton, 2001). Evidence-based practice has resulted in a quiet nursing revolution in the management and prevention of leg ulceration in community settings (Moffat *et al*, 1992). The growth of nursing knowledge and experience has supported the creation of specialist tissue viability roles that have in turn supported evidence-based leg ulcer care. King (2000) describes wound care and leg ulcer management to be the 'nurses' domain'. Reflecting the shift, GPs now often refer patients to the nurse for assessment and hosiery measurement. Although it may be the nurse who completes the assessment and makes the prescribing decision, unless he/she is a prescriber, the signature of the GP is required to authorise the prescription.

In her first report of the advisory group on nurse prescribing (Department of Health [DoH], 1989), June Crown described this practice as 'undesirable' and went on to suggest that the individual responsible for the clinical treatment decisions should also be responsible for the prescription of items required for that treatment plan. That report laid the foundation for limited eligibility to prescribe. Lord Hunt (DoH, 2001a) recently announced the intention of government to extend prescribing status to other groups of nurses but there are many who will still feel they have been left out. It is disappointing that not all nurses responsible for clinical treatment decisions within leg ulcer management and wound care presently have the right to prescribe.

Nurses with the authority to prescribe have the autonomy to assess these patients/clients and prescribe as part of a plan of care from a limited range of medicines listed in the *Nurse Prescribers' Formulary 1999–2001* (*NPF*) (Mehta, 1999). Compression or 'elastic hosiery' items are included in Appendix 8 of the *NPF* and the *British National Formulary* (*BNF*) (Mehta, 2001), and although the formulary itself is limited, there are no restrictions to the hosiery items available on NHS prescription open to the nurse prescriber (Mehta, 1999). The method chosen to supply the patient with hosiery may vary but whether the nurse is prescribing, recommending or supplying the hosiery under a patient group direction, the nurse is accountable for his/her actions and must assess each patient individually and agree a plan of care.

The nurse involved in the assessment and treatment of patients with venous disease should have an understanding of circulation to the lower limb. The knowledge will support an effective treatment decision and enable the nurse to discuss with the patient the rationale supporting treatment choice.

Physiology

Blood is supplied to the lower limbs by the anterior and posterior tibial arteries and is returned through the long and short saphenous veins and the anterior and posterior tibial veins. The anterior and posterior tibial veins lie deep in the muscle and are connected to the more superficial long and short saphenous veins by perforating or communicating veins. The veins of the lower limb have one-way bicuspid valves that close to prevent blood flow backwards towards the feet. It is the action of the valves in simultaneous conjunction with the respiratory and calf muscle pumps that affect the efficient return of venous blood from the lower limbs.

The respiratory pump

The respiratory pump aids the return of venous blood to the heart by pressure changes in the thoracic cavity. As we breathe in, the pressure within the thoracic cavity is reduced and the lungs begin to fill with air. Lower pressure in the thoracic cavity forces blood from the small peripheral vessels towards the superficial and deep veins that carry it towards the vena cava. During this phase the valves in the veins will open to allow blood to flow away from the lower limbs.

The reverse occurs as thoracic pressure increases when air is exhaled from the lungs. Higher pressures in the thoracic cavity forces venous blood towards the heart into the right atrium. Valves in the lower limb veins will close to prevent the flow of blood back towards the feet.

The calf muscle pump

The calf muscle pump also affects the efficient return of venous blood back to the heart. Venous blood in the lower limb returns by the long and short saphenous veins through adjoining perforator veins to the deep popliteal and femoral veins. Contraction of the calf muscle, while walking or moving the foot, exerts pressure on the deep anterior and posterior tibial veins that join to form the popliteal vein at the knee. The contraction and relaxation of the calf muscle forces venous return from the deep veins allowing venous blood to flow from the superficial long and short saphenous veins into the deeper veins through the perforating veins. As the muscle contracts the valves distal to the contraction close to prevent backflow while those above open to propel blood back towards the heart. As the muscle relaxes the pressure within the vein is reduced and the open valves will close again.

The development of venous hypertension

If the action of the bicuspid valves, respiratory pump or calf muscle pump is affected by inactivity or damage, venous return is compromised. An excess volume of blood will remain in the deep and superficial veins and the pressure within the vessels and surrounding tissue will increase. The perforator and superficial veins are particularly vulnerable to the pressure increase and quickly become distended and engorged with blood. Sustained pressure increase will result in venous hypertension, a condition that without treatment will soon become chronic. During venous hypertension, abnormally high pressures are transmitted to the capillary system when valve failure allows reverse blood flow (Moffat and O'Hare, 1995). Skin pigmentation, oedema, ankle flare, eczema and frequently ulceration are characteristic signs of venous hypertension.

In order to treat and prevent this condition the restoration of efficient venous return is necessary. A pressure of 30–40mmHg at the ankle reducing to 15–20mmHg just below the knee is required to achieve this aim (Morison and Moffat, 1994). Elastic or compression hosiery is manufactured to exert graduated pressure to the lower limb. It provides support to the superficial venous system and increases the efficiency of any calf muscle pump contribution. As the compression effect of the hosiery affects both venous and arterial vessels it is vital that the status of arterial circulation is determined before treatment commences.

Patient assessment

A full holistic assessment to determine the nursing, medical and social needs of the patient should precede a decision to prescribe compression hosiery. Although the Royal College of Nursing Institute (RCNI) guidelines (1998) do not go as far as identifying in detail as to what constitutes adequate training to undertake leg ulcer assessment, they do make the essential point that 'the person conducting the assessment must be trained and experienced in leg ulcer care'.

The patient's past and present medical history must be determined to identify the presence of any underlying arterial disease. A history of stroke, transient ischaemic attacks, angina or myocardial infarction has been reported to increase the probability of arterial impairment of the lower limb (Callam *et al*, 1987). Cullum and Roe (1995) also suggest that caution must be exercised if the patient has diabetes or rheumatoid arthritis, as these conditions may reduce arterial flow through the peripheral circulation. Bearing this in mind, it is interesting to note that the *NPF*, the *BNF* and the *Drug Tariff* all fail to identify arterial impairment as a caution to the prescribing of compression hosiery.

A Doppler ultrasound should be part of the holistic assessment for these patients and must be performed before compression hosiery is prescribed. Bradley (2001) has suggested that less thought is given to ascertaining the vascular status of patients who require compression hosiery as it is widely believed to exert a lower pressure than compression bandages. This is an inaccurate belief: class 3 hosiery is designed to exert a pressure equal to a high-pressure compression bandage (DoH, 2001).

A resting pressure index of 0.8 or less is widely quoted as the definitive point below which compression may compromise arterial flow (Blair *et al*, 1988; Cornwall, 1991). Bradley (2001) identifies that although this figure has been adopted in clinical practice there is a lack of research to support it. The RCNI (1998) guidelines suggest that if the resting pressure index is 0.8 or below the nurse should have specialist knowledge in order to apply and monitor the patient.

Holistic reassessment including Doppler ultrasound is required throughout the treatment period to identify the development of any factors that may contraindicate the use of compression. As the effects of graduated compression do not remain once hosicry or bandages are removed the treatment needs to be maintained through life. The longevity of treatment requires the nurse to ensure that compression hosiery remains the best treatment option for the patient and inform the patient about any new products or treatments available.

The majority of patients receive a prescription for two pairs of hosiery which, worn daily, should be replaced after six months (Cullum and Roe, 1995). The RCNI guidelines (1998) suggest that Doppler testing should be repeated at three-monthly intervals. However, anecdotal evidence suggests that many clinics have found themselves unable to cope with the number of patients requiring reassessment and Doppler so frequently. Considering the lack of substantial evidence to support three-monthly reassessment, many clinics reassess at six-monthly intervals while asking the patients to contact them earlier if there are any concerns (Jones and Nelson, 1998). The timing also coincides with the need for a new hosiery prescription.

The psychological implications involved in wearing compression hosiery are not often considered, as the patient is 'expected to comply' with treatment. The initial assessment provides an ideal opportunity to explore the patient's perception, attitude, ability and motivation to wear continuously compression hosiery. The concept of concordance — in preference to compliance or adherence to medication regimes — underpins the education of nurse prescribers. While compliance indicates the patient should comply with instructions, adherence suggests the patient will stick to the agreed plan. Concordance is a concept described by the National Prescribing Centre (1998) as the equal partnership of patient and prescriber during the negotiation of treatment options. Achieving this aim may appear idealistic but the longevity of treatment requires an approach that will optimise both the cost effectiveness and clinical outcomes of care.

Classification of compression hosiery

Graduated compression hosiery is produced in three classifications, reflecting the pressure in millimetres of mercury exerted by the garment at the ankle (*Table 8.1*). Each classification is listed with the indications for use.

Table 8.1: Classes of compression hosiery

Class	Compression (mmHg)	Indications for use
1	14–17	Light support. Superficial or early carices. Varicosis during pregnancy
2	18–24	Medium support. Varices of medium severity. Ulcer treatment and prophylaxis. Mild oedema. Varicosis during pregnancy
3	25–39	Strong support. Gross varices, post-thrombotic venous insufficiency. Gross oedema, ulcer treatment and prophylaxis

Source: Mehta, 1999; DoH, 2001b

Limb measurement

The importance of accurate assessment cannot be overemphasised, but once the decision has been taken to supply hosiery, accurate measurement is paramount. Pressure exerted from an ill-fitting garment can either be insufficient to create a therapeutic effect or too great, possibly causing tissue damage. Moffat and O'Hare (1995) identified six common sites at risk of tissue damage:

- tibial crest
- constricting cuffs around the knees
- dorsum of the foot
- ankle deformity
- crowded and deformed toes
- bunion area.

The common element in these risk areas is the close proximity of bone to the surface of the skin. In contrast to compression bandages, hosiery garments are applied in direct contact with the surface of the skin. There is no padding layer to protect these vulnerable areas.

As identified in the introduction, the pharmacist may take the measurements and advise the patient with the choice of product. Although he/she may be able and willing to take the measurements, it can be argued that a busy pharmacy does not afford the private space required to maintain the patient's dignity while measurements are taken. Dressings, bandages and hosiery should be removed before each leg is measured individually. The optimum time to measure the leg for hosiery is early in the morning before the limb is dependent or following a period of at least one hour's elevated rest (O'Hare, 1997; Courtenay and Butler, 1999). O'Hare (1997) identified that patients who are measured for thigh-length garments should be standing during measurement. Although O'Hare did not identify the need to adopt this position for below-knee hosiery measurements, it is easier to accurately measure the leg when the patient is standing (Edwards, 1999).

Evidence to support the points from which the leg measurements should be taken vary, but Scholl (1996) and Cullum and Roe (1995) offered some consistency with the following list:

- the leg circumference at the narrowest point of the ankle
- the leg circumference at the widest point of the calf
- the circumference of the middle thigh (for thigh-length hosiery).

Scholl (1996) also suggested that measurements should be taken from the heel to the toe. This measurement is necessary to establish the fitting of closed-toe hosiery. A wipe-clean or disposable tape measure should be used to prevent cross-infection. The tape should not be twisted or be pulled tight around the leg during measurement. If any one of the measurements taken does not fall within the product size specifications for ready-made hosiery on either leg, made-to-measure hosiery must be prescribed. It is important that comparisons are not made between the sizes of different companies; for example, the calf measurement for a medium size below-knee sock by one manufacturer may fall into the large size sock measurement for another manufacturer.

Made-to-measure products require that additional measurements are taken and are available in knee and thigh length. Each manufacturer has a specific form that must be completed in order to obtain made-to-measure hosiery. The forms have a picture identifying the points of measurement required and a chart into which the measurements are entered. They can be obtained from the pharmacist or directly from the hosiery company. Using the measurements provided, hosiery is custom-made for each limb.

Patients who pay for their prescriptions will pay the prescription fee for each hosiery garment rather than one fee for the pair. Hosiery garment prices are listed in the *Drug Tariff*. Items range in price from £6.00 for some ready-made items to £32.60 (DoH, 2001b) for made-to-measure hosiery. The price listed in the *Drug Tariff* refers to the NHS cost for a pair of hosiery garments.

Product range

There is a wide range of hosiery products available. Although the choice of product can rely on the patient's preference and need in relation to the assessment, not all choices are available in all classifications in any one product range. Open-toe garments are preferred by some patients and can be useful when fitting patients with large feet or for those who are unable to remove their own hosiery as access to the toes is possible. As there is little evidence to suggest a therapeutic advantage between knee or thigh-length hosiery (Moffatt and O'Hare, 1995), the patient can make the choice. Anecdotal evidence suggests that most patients prefer below-knee hosiery although there are still some female patients who prefer thigh-length garments they can attach to their suspender belt. Cosmetic appearance can be very important to both male and female patients. Colour options vary depending on the manufacturer's range and the popularity of the item, but items may be available in black, brown, honey and sand colours, though the actual colour will vary according to the fabric used. Men sometimes prefer black, brown or navy colours produced in a sock with a 'rib' appearance.

Sensitisation is a problem experienced by some patients; Moffat and Dorman (1995) described how erythema and itching may result from contact with lycra. Cullum and Roe (1995) also identified elastodiene, rubber, nylon and elastane used in the manufacture of hosiery products to be common causes of sensitivity. Patients who experience sensitisation may find a cotton liner applied under the stocking helpful (O'Hare, 1997), or may opt for a cotton rich hosiery product. These products are not 100% cotton and are only available in class 11 mid-tan colour at present, but they are reported in local clinics to be well tolerated by patients.

Application advice

Patients with limited dexterity may require help to apply their hosiery. The involvement of family carers, or a social services referral is sometimes necessary. Class 1 and 2 hosiery are generally easier to apply as they are thinner but they may not exert the required amount of pressure to the limb. The pressure exerted by hosiery is cumulative, so two class 1 hosiery items worn on the same limb will exert a pressure equal to that of a single class 2 garment. Although not recommended, this may be an option (Moffatt and O'Hare, 1995). Patients frequently find hosiery difficult to apply (Morison and Moffat, 1994) so many use inventive techniques to help them (eg. rubber gloves to maximise finger grip). There are two main methods to ease hosiery application.

A hosiery applicator can be purchased to help patients who find it difficult to reach their toes. This is a frame with outer handles and an inner column.

❖ The hosiery garment is applied to the centre column of the applicator.

❖ Once applied the toe section of the garment lies open allowing the patient to place the foot into it.

❖ The limb is lowered into the applicator as the frame is gently pulled upwards.

Patients who prefer open-toe hosiery may find the silk half-sock supplied by some manufacturers useful:

- the sock is applied to the toe and foot before the hosiery
- the hosiery garment slides easily over the silk material
- the foot section is applied and care should be taken to ensure the heel is correctly positioned
- the length of the garment is then gently pulled up the limb
- the silk half-sock is then pulled out of the end of the stocking.

Hosiery care

It is important that the patient is aware how to care for their hosiery. A leaflet inside each pack of hosiery will give the patient specific care instructions. Washing and emollient preparations will adversely affect the elasticity of the product and subsequently the pressure exerted by the hosiery. Manufacturers usually state that hosiery should be hand-washed in warm soapy water and dried away from heat or sunlight. Patients are advised, if possible, to apply emollients overnight when hosiery is removed to prevent hosiery damage. This is not always possible as some patients require assistance and as a result may only remove the garments on a weekly basis. If hosiery is reapplied soon after emollients have been applied to the skin, it will be necessary to monitor the elasticity of the hosiery and reorder more frequently.

Conclusion

Although evidence to support the effectiveness of compression hosiery is sparse, many practitioners agree it is the most effective tool in the prevention of recurrent ulceration (Moffat and Harper, 1997). The depth of knowledge held by many nurses has placed them in an effective position to assess, treat and evaluate the use of compression hosiery. Although compliance to compression hosiery regimes is problematic, the nurse working in partnership with the patient will promote the opportunity for cost-effective and therapeutically effective care.

Key Points

※ The patient must be individually assessed to ascertain suitability for compression therapy.

※ Accurate measurements must be taken from specific points of the leg.

※ Size parameters vary for each manufacturer.

※ Never 'make do' with a size. If the measurements do not match, made-to-measure hosiery must be prescribed.

※ Reassess the patient at regular intervals to ensure compression hosiery remains the best treatment option for the patient.

References

Blair SD, Wright DDI, Backhouse CD (1988) Sustained compression and healing of chronic venous ulcers. *Br Med J* **297**: 1159–61

Bradley L (2001) Venous haemodynamics and the effects of compression stockings. *Br J Community Nurs* **6**(4): 165–75

Callam MJ, Harper DR, Dale J, Ruckley CV (1987) Chronic ulcer of the leg. *Br Med J* **294**: 1389–91

Cornwall J (1991) Managing venous leg ulcers. *Community Outlook* May: 36–8

Courtenay M, Butler M (1999) *Nurse Prescribing Principles and Practice*. Greenwich Medical Media, London

Cullum N, Roe B (1995) *Leg Ulcers: Nursing Management. A Research-Based Guide*. Ballière Tindall, London

Department of Health (1989) *Report of the Advisory Group on Nurse Prescribing* (Chair: Crown J). DoH, London

Department of Health (2001a) *Patients Get Quicker Access to Medicines*. Press release, May 4th 2001/0223

Department of Health (2001b) *Drug Tariff*. The Stationery Office, London

Edwards L (1999) Preventing the recurrence of venous leg ulceration. *J Community Nurs* **13**(11): 35–40

Jones JE, Nelson EA (1998) Compression hosiery in the management of venous leg ulcers. *J Wound Care* **7**(6): 293–6

King B (2000) Prescribing: The role of the tissue viability nurse. *Nurs Times Plus* Sept: 19–20

Mehta D, ed (1999) *Nurse Prescribers' Formulary*. British Medical Association/Royal Pharmaceutical Society of Great Britain, London

Mehta D, ed (2001) *British National Formulary 41*. British Medical Association/Royal Pharmaceutical Society of Great Britain, London

Mishton A (2001) The continuing education programme. Module 33: compression hosiery. *Pharmacy Magazine*. http://www.pharmacymag.co.uk/module33.html (accessed 25 June 2001)

Moffat CJ, Dorman MC (1995) Recurrance of leg ulcers within a community ulcer service. *J Wound Care* **4**(2): 57–61

Moffat CJ, Franks PJ, Oldroyd M *et al* (1992) Community clinics for leg ulcers and impacts on healing. *Br Med J* **305**: 1389–92

Moffat M, Harper P (1997) *Leg Ulcers*. Churchill Livingstone, London

Moffat M, O'Hare L (1995) Graduated compression hosiery for venous ulceration. *J Wound Care* **4**(10): 459–62

Morison M, Moffat C (1994) *A Colour Guide to the Assessment and Management of Leg Ulcers*. 2nd edn. Mosby, London

National Prescribing Centre (1998) *Nurse Prescribing Resource Pack: Signposts for Prescribing Nurses — Principles of Good Prescribing*. National Prescribing Centre, Liverpool

O'Hare L (1997) Scholl compression hosiery in the management of venous disorders. *Br J Nurs* **6**(7): 391–4

Royal College of Nursing Institute (1998) *Clinical Practice Guidelines: The Management of Patients with Venous Leg Ulcers. Technical report*. Royal College of Nursing Institute, University of York, York

Scholl (1996) *The Complete Guide to Healthcare for Legs*. Scholl, Luton

9

The patient's view: the benefits and limitations of nurse prescribing

N Brooks, C Otway, C Rashid, E Kilty, C Maggs

This study was undertaken in a primary care group to explore nurse prescribing from the patient/client's viewpoint. All prescribing health visitors, district nurses and practice nurses were asked to recruit five patients for whom they had prescribed; fifty patients/clients participated in the study. Identified benefits of nurse prescribing included a more effective use of the nurse's and doctor's time; a quality relationship between the nurse and patient; nurses' awareness of their own professional limitations; their expertise in certain types of care; and their providing timely, convenient, practical and successful treatment. Limitations and the proposed options for change included the training and competency of nurse prescribers and the limitations of the Nurse Prescribers' Formulary. On a local level the study informs nurse prescribers that they are currently meeting the needs of the majority of recipients, and provides evidence of some of the benefits and limitations of nurse prescribing.

Nurse prescribing could be seen as one of the most significant changes to take place in nursing as a response to patient need identified in the Cumberlege Report (Department of Health and Social Security [DHSS], 1986). From October 1994, district nurses, health visitors and practice nurses have been able to prescribe. The significance of this was not the number of nurses affected (as this was relatively small compared with the whole nursing workforce), but the fact that it overturned traditional professional boundaries whereby doctors prescribed, pharmacists dispensed and nurses administered (Department of Health [DoH], 1989).

Since Luker *et al*'s demonstration project of 1994 (1997a, b; 1998), there has been little research exploring nurse prescribing from the patient/client perspective. Following searches on Medline, CINAHL, British Nursing Index and the National Research Register, the authors were unable to find any such published research. The need for such research is even more important in light of the *Review of Prescribing, Supply and Administration of Medicines* (DoH, 1999) and the consultation paper (DoH, 2000a) inviting professionals to consider the issues surrounding nurse prescribing. These include the principles of nurse prescribing, extending the *Nurse Prescribers' Formulary* (*NPF*), and which groups of nurses should be selected to undertake preparation and training. One of the intentions of this consultation is that patient need should govern any extension to nurse prescribing authority (DoH, 2000a).

This chapter will present part of a study undertaken from May to September 2000, which explored nurse prescribing from the patient/client's perspective.

Literature review

Patient evaluation of nurse prescribing has centred on the demonstration project of 1994 (Luker *et al*, 1997b) that evaluated the social, emotional and financial benefits to the patient and/or carer. It was conducted in the early phase of nurse prescribing when nurses had just qualified and were new to the role. In general, patients considered nurses to have sufficient knowledge to prescribe the items included in the *NPF*, and that in some instances nurses were in a better position than doctors to prescribe because of their knowledge, eg. in areas such as wound care.

Saving time for GPs, as well as patients, was identified as a further benefit of nurse prescribing, along with appropriate use of time. Patients did not have to make appointments to see GPs or see them about what they perceived to be relatively minor problems. In addition, nurses could prescribe items quicker, meaning treatment could be initiated sooner.

The patients identified that nurse prescribers were more approachable and more time was spent in consultation with them. Satisfaction with this consultation process centred around the fact that nurses 'spoke the same language,' ie. they used less medical jargon. Nurse consultations were more relaxed, possibly because prescribing often occurred in the patients' homes rather than at GP practices. In Luker *et al*'s (1997b) study, 13% of patients reported that nurses provided them with better information than GPs. This satisfaction was increased by the fact that nurses were perceived to be more aware of patients' personal circumstances.

More than half of the patients in the study reported seeking a consultation with the nurse in preference to the GP. This did not appear to be related to the nurse prescribing role (Luker *et al*, 1998); the main reasons given were convenience and preference, based on previous experiences. It could be argued that the issue of nurse prescribing might have been overshadowed in the reasons for consultation. Patients identified nurse prescribing as more convenient because they did not have to make an appointment to see the GP — which for non-urgent conditions could take several days or weeks — and nurse prescribers offered alternative systems. For example, as well as visiting mothers at home, health visitors provided drop-in clinics.

Very few disadvantages to nurse prescribing were identified. Initially there was confusion over what could be prescribed, however, Luker *et al* (1997a) reported that patients became familiar with this and were clear in their own minds about the professional boundaries between the nurse and GP regarding what could be prescribed by whom. Patients who required medication on prescription as well as items from the *NPF*, eg. catheter products and dressings, identified a further disadvantage: previously both had been contained in one prescription whereas under the new system, GPs and nurses prescribed separately. The same issue arose with item delivery — some nurses had previously delivered nursing and medical items, but with the new system they only brought the items that they had prescribed. In some instances, therefore, the onus to obtain the medication prescribed by the GP was transferred to the patient.

Methodologically, there may have been some limitations with *et al*'s (1997b) study. Alderman (1996), a community nurse involved in the demonstration project, found that completing the patient diaries that formed part of the evaluation was problematic for some of the older patients. Although semi-structured interviews were also carried out, the diaries formed a substantive part of the evaluation; difficulty completing them might have limited the richness of the data collected.

Study design

For the present study, a qualitative, descriptive design was chosen, as its conditions were most appropriate to the needs of this study. This design lends itself to the discovery of new facts about a situation

(Leninger, 1985; Brink and Wood, 1991; Cormack, 1996). The descriptive design was inductive in order to build on existing theory concerning nurse prescribing. A further consideration for adopting this design was to ensure that the patients' views of nurse prescribing were captured rather than the anticipated views of the steering group.

Registration and ethics

The project was registered with the trust, and ethical approval obtained from the university and area health authority ethics committee. Consent from the primary care group (PCG) was obtained through the PCG board nurse who was also a member of the steering group.

The setting

This study was undertaken in one PCG in Leicestershire and the local trust had commenced its nurse prescribing training programme more than three years previously. Unlike the demonstration project of 1994 (Luker *et al*, 1997b), the nurse prescribers in this study were experienced. The study was conducted in the Blaby and Lutterworth PCG which has a population of approximately 94,000, of which 97% is white. Unemployment in the area is low — 4.4% against a county figure of 7.5% (Blaby and Lutterworth PCG, 2000). The majority of the population falls between the ages of twenty-five and fifty-nine years and 15% of the population live more than three miles from their GP practice (Blaby and Lutterworth PCG, 2000).

Recruitment

All prescribing health visitors (n=17), district nurses (n=9) and practice nurses (n=1) in the PCG were informed of the study and their participation requested at team meetings. They were asked to recruit and gain informal consent for five of the most recent patients for whom they had prescribed (total population size, n=135). The contact details of these patients were given to the steering group, of which three members obtained formal consent and undertook data collection.

In total fifty-four patients were recruited, of whom fifty consented to participation and took part in an interview. Four patients were not interviewed due to ill-health, failure to reply to interview dates issued through the post and one patient's holiday coinciding with the data collection period. Recruitment was not as expected despite the nurse prescribers expressing enthusiasm before the study began and being kept informed of its progress. Only five nurse prescribers were able to recruit five patients, so an anonymous letter was sent after the data collection period to identify why the predicted numbers had not been achieved. The two main reasons identified were nurse prescribers not needing to write five prescriptions and not having time to recruit participants because of heavy workloads.

Although the demographics of the participants were not specifically recorded, some characteristics could be identified. Some participants offered information on how often they used the nurse prescribing service: 68% of those that offered this information were classified as low or new users of nurse prescribers as they had only received between one and three prescriptions. The participants ranged from mothers of under-fives who were in their twenties and thirties, to older people in their eighties; all were white and spoke English as their first language.

Methodology

To identify the patients' experiences of nurse prescribing in order to contribute to nursing science and practice, issues were specifically explored regarding:

- patients' reactions to/experiences of nurse prescribing
- acceptability of current practice
- patient benefits, eg. reducing under-reporting of minor symptoms, increased compliance with treatment, knowledge gains, a more patient-centred/holistic approach
- limitations or inconveniences.

This chapter will report on the issues of patient/client benefits and limitations of nurse prescribing.

Developing the interview schedule

The steering group developed four interview questions, based on the literature and the aims of the study. These were:

- could you please share with me your experiences of nurse prescribing?
- how do you feel about nurses being able to prescribe?
- do you feel there were any gains/benefits for you by the nurse being able to prescribe?
- do you feel that there were any disadvantages/ inconveniences for you by the nurse being able to prescribe?

The questions were not piloted prior to the interviews as they were considered to be straightforward. They were broad so that the participants could relay their experiences in their own words. The three members of the steering group who undertook the interviews however, did agree on prompts that would be used if patients required examples. For example, advantages of nurse prescribing might be convenience, approachability etc. These prompts were based on the findings of Luker *et al* (1997b).

Data collection

Data were collected by interviews which were conducted either face-to-face in the participants' homes or over the telephone. Organised at each participant's convenience, they provided the opportunity for a prepared explanation of the research as well as time to answer any questions. This may have contributed to the high participation levels (Oppenheim, 1992).

Data analysis

Qualitative data was generated from the interviews and analysed according to content theme analysis (Burnard, 1991). This is a form of content analysis in which raw data from initial categories are grouped to form mutually exclusive categories. Quantitative data was applied during the analysis phase to identify the size of the responses. The use of independent checking by three members of the group was employed to validate the results that were generated from the data. The themes developed from the data were compared for consistency and consensus was achieved.

Sandelowski (1986) stated that the typical and atypical elements of the data should be included in order to maintain rigour and validity in qualitative research. Taking this into consideration, all of the interview data was incorporated into themes and included in the results.

Results

The findings from this study confirm the majority of the anticipated benefits of nurse prescribing identified in the Crown Report (DoH, 1989) and some of the findings of the demonstration project of 1994 (Luker *et al*, 1997b). However, the findings of this study relate to nurse prescribers who are more experienced. Therefore, unlike Luker *et al*'s (1997b) study, nurse prescribing could be explored as a separate entity in more detail. Also, unlike Luker *et al*'s (1997b) study, the participants were not all high users of the nurse prescribing service and had not been in regular contact with the nurses over a period of time. As the participants in this study were low, new and intermittent users, these results could be considered as relatively uninfluenced by the continuing relationship between themselves and the nurse and the services that the nurse provided for them.

Effective use of nurses' and doctors' time

The participants identified several benefits of nurse prescribing: 46% commented that nurse prescribing demonstrated better use of the GPs' and nurses' time. Patients recognised that GPs were busy and that the more 'minor' problems were best dealt with by a nurse prescriber leaving the GP free to deal with more 'serious' problems:

> *Saved time also for the doctor because the [health visitor] had diagnosed the condition and was able to prescribe.*

(Participant 11)

> *It's more effective use of the nurse's time.*

(Participant 19)

What the participants identified appeared to reflect the intentions of *The NHS Plan* (DoH, 2000b); namely, to support the renegotiation of roles in order to maximise the talents of the NHS workforce.

Nurse prescribers, like the nurse practitioner, have taken on roles that were previously exclusive to the medical domain (NHS Management Executive, 1993). The practical application of this change in roles was supported by the participants, something which Chapple *et al* (2000) considered to be instrumental in the extent to which these new roles gain legitimacy.

Awareness of professional limitations

The participants identified that nurse prescribers' awareness of their professional limitations was also an advantage:

> *If the health visitor is not happy with your problem she recognises her limitations and has even gone and made me a doctor's appointment.*

(Participant 1)

It appeared that some of the nurse prescribers made the patients aware of what they could, and could not, do. If treating a problem was beyond their expertise, they then gave appropriate advice recommending that patients go to see their GPs. These findings are pertinent in light of the nurse prescribing consultation paper (DoH, 2000), because although there is the potential for nurses to prescribe more, they need to show that they will prescribe with due care. One of the options in the consultation document (option 5) proposed extending prescribing rights to include all general sales list (GSL), pharmacy-only (P), and all licensed prescription-only medicines (PoMs). This option proposed that, like dentists and doctors, nurses would use their professional judgement to decide which medicines patients need, and would be competent to prescribe. Some of the participants in this study identified that this already occurred with a limited nurse prescribing formulary, and therefore would be likely to continue regardless of the range of medicines to which nurse prescribers would have access.

Expertise of nurse prescribers

Some of the participants identified the expertise of the nurse prescriber as a further benefit. Nurse prescribers were seen as experts in wound care, catheter care, nappy rash, mastitis, thrush, common complaints in mothers and babies, eg. feeding or sleep problems, and dry skin/eczema. They were deemed to be experts as they dealt with the problems regularly, were knowledgeable, practical and provided alternatives if the original treatment failed to work.

Timeliness

Seventy-two per cent of the participants identified timeliness of treatment as a benefit. They liked the responsiveness to their particular need, and the majority of participants usually got an assessment by the nurse and a prescription in the same day. One participant noted that it was:

> *The only thing that has been quick in my experience of the NHS.*

> (Participant 7)

This also meant that participants were able to start their treatment sooner:

> *With the nurse prescribing straight away I got two doses in on the first day rather than waiting to see the GP the next day, which was good as it may have got worse while I was waiting.*

> (Participant 24)

Nurse prescribing is currently limited to minor treatments, so whether all participants' treatments needed to start straight away and whether some ailments might have improved without a prescription could be questioned. Cost benefits in this instance will probably be emotive, balancing individual needs against what is effective. However in this case, timeliness of treatment demonstrates evidence of flexible ways of working to providing better services for patients, as outlined in *The NHS Plan* (DoH, 2000b).

Convenience

Forty-six per cent of the participants identified nurse prescribing as more convenient. This included not having to make a physical trip to the GP practice and having care and treatment centred on their needs in their own homes. This relatively new method of service delivery appears to highlight the inefficiencies of the previous system:

> *In the past she has said what has been wrong, she confirms what it is and I go to the GP because she can't prescribe it and he says the same.*

(Participant 8)

Practicality of the nurse prescriber

A further benefit identified was the practical nature of the nurse prescriber. The participants identified how the nurse prescribers knew the system and best methods of delivery to make sure that they got the most from the prescription:

> *The nurse also arranged the prescription as I had the wrong bag when I came out of hospital. She called the chemist at 6.00 pm and the bags were ready to be collected first thing in the morning.*

(Participant 4)

> *The health visitor prescribed treatment for oral thrush and eye ointment. The eye ointment worked, the oral thrush medication didn't as the chemist dispensed a spoon and not a pipette and the baby spat it out. The health visitor thought this might happen so came back and prescribed something else which worked.*

(Participant 41)

This aspect of nurse prescribing was identified by Mallison (1984), who claimed that the practical nature of nurses was due to positive interpersonal skills which enabled them to make the system work by resolving and working around problems such as wound healing or skin care. Another aspect, not identified by Mallison, may be that of experience. The nurse prescribers in this study were working in a trust which had started its training programme three years previously and therefore the practical nature of the nurse prescribers may have also been due to the 'hands-on' experience of prescribing similar drugs.

Nurse–patient relationship

The participants identified the quality of the nurse prescribers' relationship with them as a further benefit. This was characterised by the nurse providing reassurance, continuity of care, information and health promotion details, and being approachable. One participant stated that:

> *It's easier to build a rapport with the nurse as doctors are always so busy.*

> (Participant 32)

The relationship took the form of a 'consultancy' with the nurse, due to her knowledge and clinical experience being able to command authority. Humphris (1994) identified the benefits of this process whereby the consultant acts as initiator and the recipient is free to accept or reject the recommendations. As one of the participants noted:

> *At the end of the day it's the patient's choice — they can always visit the GP if they are not happy with the [health visitor's] prescription.*

> (Participant 36)

Continuity of care

Continuity of care was highlighted as a significant part of the role of the nurse prescriber:

> *The [health visitor] knows your baby since they were tiny and so it's better than going to see the GP especially when it's a big practice.*

> (Participant 2)

Chapple *et al* (2000) have identified this as central to satisfaction with nurse-led services. They noted that:

> *The re-establishment of social support and continuity of care by the nurse-led service provided the basis for high*

> *levels of satisfaction and confidence in the role of the nurse as the principle provider of primary care.*

Participants also valued being given information on health promotion or practical advice about the prescription. This had been identified by Luker *et al* (1997b). This type of approach may have increased compliance with treatment or equipped patients with the information to be able to care for themselves and thereby control, or manage, the treatment for which the prescription was issued. Participants commented that:

> *I have been given several prescriptions for my son's eczema and I have also been given lots of background information.*

> (Participant 10)

> *She also went through all the things that may have caused my baby's itchy skin like a new baby bath or washing powder.*

> (Participant 16)

This good quality relationship identified by some of the participants may have been instrumental in addressing the issue of under-reporting:

> *With the [health visitor] you talk things over with them and you don't feel such an idiot.*

> (Participant 1)

> *She is more approachable and I don't mind phoning her, unlike the GP.*

> (Participant 8)

This reluctance of patients to inform doctors of what they perceive to be minor issues has long been recognised within the medical profession (Cartwright and Smith, 1988).

Future improvements

The findings from this study provide evidence that nurse prescribers were successfully meeting the needs of the patients/clients. Of the fifty participants, forty-nine (98%) were happy with the nurse prescribing process, which included consultation and discussion regarding the effect of the prescription in remedying the problem. The remaining participant had misunderstood the role of the district nurse, and thought she would be given her prescribed items at the time of prescription and would not have to collect them from the chemist. This study may partly redress the paucity of evidence regarding the quality of patient consultations and outcomes, as identified by Rees and Kinnersley (1996).

The participants finally reflected on the limitations of the system at that time and anticipated changes to nurse prescribing. Thirty-three (66%) were happy with nurse prescribing and unable to identify either disadvantages or areas for improvement. This was positive in affirming that nurse prescribing was meeting the needs of these recipients. The remaining seventeen (34%) identified areas for further nurse prescribing rights which, in their view, would make the service more efficient. It is worth noting here that 68% of the participants were new or low users (1–3 prescriptions) and the participants who suggested the need for further prescribing rights tended to be those who had more experience of this service. This appears to reflect Hart's (1996) view that there is a growing body of knowledge, suggesting that patients who have repeated exposure to healthcare services become more informed and critical of the services provided.

The areas identified by these participants in which nurse prescribing could be further expanded included providing repeat prescriptions and prescribing from a wider formulary — particularly with regard to oral medications and those for the under-fives:

> *I wish the nurse could prescribe antibiotics, as I had to wait two days to see the doctor for an infected wound before I could get them.*

> (Participant 22)

> *... when my baby was only two weeks old I got mastitis, the [health visitor] knew what it was, I didn't. She said I needed antibiotics but couldn't prescribe them, so I had to go with the baby down to the doctor's. It was hard battling with the receptionist even though I told her that the [health visitor] said I should be seen that day. I eventually saw the GP and was given antibiotics but it would have been much easier if I could have been prescribed them by the [health visitor].*

> (Participant 29)

The key word used by these participants when they talked about extending nurse prescribing was 'continuity'. The nurses were seen as instrumental in carrying on the work of prescribing rather than prescribing independently. This reflects the role of the 'dependent prescriber' (DoH, 1999) in which prescribers will be authorised to prescribe certain medication for patients whose condition has already been assessed by an independent prescriber. Shepperd (1998) reflected similar sentiments, stating that collaborative frameworks might be more beneficial as nurses could work in partnership with doctors and pharmacists to make treatment decisions.

Training issues

Twenty-six per cent of participants highlighted training issues in relation to justification for and against further expansion to nurse prescribing. They recognised that medical training equipped doctors to prescribe without any restrictions, unlike nurses who would need to undertake further training if they were to extend prescribing rights at a later date:

> *I am happy for the nurse to prescribe medication for the baby as long as its more simple things, complicated or serious things should be taken to the doctor... as they are trained to do this.*

(Participant 25)

> *It could go a little bit further, for example they should be able to prescribe antibiotics for ear infections as long as they have had the training.*

(Participant 30)

This recognition of nurse prescribers needing to be educated and competent is also a government concern (DoH, 1999; DoH, 2000). The Crown Report (DoH, 1999) stated that:

> *All legally prescribers should take personal responsibility for maintaining and updating their knowledge and practice relating to prescribing... and should never prescribe in situations beyond their professional competence.*

The consultation paper on nurse prescribing (DoH, 2000a) also identified the need for not only an educational preparation process, but also a robust continuing professional development programme to ensure that competence is maintained. This may not only strengthen the skills and expertise of the nurse prescriber but also public confidence. However this may take more reassurance on the nurse prescribers' part; as Luker *et al* (1997) discovered, nurses are already anxious about their diagnostic skills with the current prescribing formulary.

Limitations of the study

Two aspects of this study may have limited its generalisability. Although the approach could be applied to other user groups, the sample was a convenience one and, having identified the characteristics of the participants and the setting in which the study took place, the findings may not reflect the views of a non-white population from different socioeconomic backgrounds. In addition, the nurse prescribers undertook recruitment because patient details could not be released to the research team except by the nurse prescribers' first gaining patient consent for this to happen. The ethics committee recommended this approach to protect patient confidentiality. If the research team had been able to randomly and retrospectively select patients, this limitation could have been avoided. Although asked to recruit consecutively, to limit the possibility of nurses actively selecting patients, no controls were put in place to monitor this.

Conclusion

This study has identified the efficacy of nurse prescribing in one PCG in Leicestershire, from the user's point of view. Nurse prescribers were, in the main, meeting the needs of the participants, with positive experiences identified in terms of the prescribing process and the outcome.

The reality of nurse prescribing and suggestions for its future development made by the study participants preempted those that have recently been made by the government. These include the need for education to maintain public safety and develop and maintain competence, the potential for the *NPF* to be expanded, and the need to provide patient-centred services and renegotiate traditional roles so that the NHS workforce is used more effectively.

The government gave their commitment to nurse prescribing in 2000 with the publication of *The NHS Plan* (DoH, 2000b). Following an extended consultation period, option 3 has been declared the preferred option. In total, £10 million has been allocated to train an anticipated 10,000 nurses to prescribe. Existing nurse prescribers and new nurse prescribers will be trained to prescribe all GSL and P medicines, together with a specified range of PoMs used for certain conditions, eg. hay fever, minor injuries and palliative care. Nurse prescribers will be also able to prescribe nicotine replacement therapy. This study provides evidence to support this development as one which would meet patients needs and expectations.

Key Points

- ⌘ Patients/clients are instrumental in identifying the reality of current service provision and in proposing future changes.
- ⌘ Nurse prescribing can improve use of the nurses' and doctors' time and be more convenient and practical for patients, leading to better relationships between themselves and nurses and more successful treatment outcomes.
- ⌘ Proposed changes to nurse prescribing include training nurse prescribers.
- ⌘ Nurse prescribing in practice reflects the government philosophy of a patient-centred service, which is valued by patients and clients.

References

Alderman C (1996) Prescribing pioneers. *Nurs Standard* **10**(18): 26–7

Blaby, Lutterworth PCG (2000) *Community PCG Community Profile*. Unpublished.

Brink PJ, Wood MJ (1991) *Advanced Design in Nursing Research*. Sage Publications, London

Burnard P (1991) A method of analysing interview transcripts in qualitative research. *Nurse Educ Today* **11**(6): 461–6

Cartwright A, Smith C (1988) *Elderly People and their Medicines*. Routledge, London

Chapple A, Rogers A, Macdonald W, Sergison M (2000) Patients' perceptions of changing professional boundaries and the future of 'nurse-led services'. *Primary Health Care Research and Development* **1**(1): 51–9

Cormack DFS (1996) *The Research Process in Nursing*. 3rd edn. Blackwell Scientific Publications, Oxford

Department of Health and Social Security (1986) *Neighbourhood Nursing: A Focus for Care*. (Cumberlege Report) HMSO, London

Department of Health (1999) *Review of Prescribing, Supply and Administration of Medicines. Report on the Supply and Administration of Medicines*. HSC 1998/051. NHS E, Leeds

Department of Health (1989) *Report of the Advisory Group on Nurse Prescribing*. (Crown Report). DoH, London

Department of Health (2000a) *Consultation on Proposals to Extend Nurse Prescribing*. Accessed November 2000. http://www.doh.gov.uk/nurseprescribing

Department of Health (2000b) *The NHS Plan. A Plan for Investment. A Plan for Reform*. CM4818I. The Stationery Office, London

Hart M (1996) Incorporating outpatient perceptions into definitions of quality. *J Adv Nurs* **24**(6): 1234–40

Humphris D (1994) *The Clinical Nurse Specialist: Issues in Practice*. Macmillan Press, London

Leninger M (1985) *Qualitative Research Methods in Nursing*. Grine and Stratton, Orlando

Luker K, Austin L, Hogg C, Ferguson B, Smith K (1997a) Patients' views of nurse prescribing. *Nurs Times* **93**(17): 51–5

Luker K, Austin L, Hogg C et al (1997b) *Evaluation of Nurse Prescribing: Final Report*. The University of Liverpool and The University of York

Luker K, Austin L, Hogg C, Ferguson B, Smith K (1998) Nurse-patient relationships: the context of nurse prescribing. *J Adv Nurs* **28**(2): 235–42

Mallison M (1984) The shoes of the clinician. *Am J Nurs* **84**(6): 587

NHS Management Executive (1993) *A Vision for the Future: The Nursing, Midwifery and Health Visiting Contribution to Health Care*. DoH, Leeds

Oppenheim P (1992) *Questionnaire Design, Interviewing and Attitude Measurement*. Pinter, New York

Rees M, Kinnersley P (1996) Nurse-led management of minor illness in a GP surgery. *Nurs Times* **92**(6): 32–3

Sandelowski M (1986) The problem of rigour in qualitative research. *Adv Nurs Sci* **8**(3): 27–37

Shepperd E (1998) I prescribe, therefore I am. *Nursing* **94**(14): 34–5

10

Nurse prescribing: views on autonomy and independence

Chris Rodden

The introduction of nurse prescribing throughout Scotland in the primary care setting has proved to be an interesting development for nurses. The aim of this study was to assess the impact of nurse prescribing on district nurses and health visitors in one NHS trust in Scotland. All prescribing nurses in the trust were asked to participate in the study. This explored their perceptions of autonomy and the level of dependence on GP colleagues since being able to prescribe. In addition, prescribing patterns were examined to ascertain whether there was a relationship between the area of nursing (eg. district nursing or health visiting) or the length of prescribing experience, and the number of prescriptions written.

The Cumberlege Report (1986) first raised the issue regarding nurses being able to prescribe. However, it was not until six years later that the necessary legislation was in place to facilitate this process — namely the Medicinal Products: Prescription by Nurses etc Act 1992. This Act set out conditions under which certain nurses would be able to prescribe from a limited formulary (National Board for Nursing, Midwifery and Health Visiting for Scotland [NBS], 1997).

At present, for nurses to prescribe within the community setting, they must possess either a district nursing or health visiting qualification. Therefore nurses with extensive knowledge and experience are participating in this development, including practice nurses with the appropriate qualifications. The government has announced their support in taking forward recommendations of the Review of Prescribing, Supply and Administration of Medicines (NHS Executive, 1999). This includes extending the scope of nurse prescribing (Scottish Executive, 2001). This will enable new groups of nurses to prescribe and also increase the items that can be prescribed by nurses.

McCartney *et al* (1999) identified three primary aims of the introduction of nurse prescribing:

- to save money
- to transfer routine medical work to nurses
- to challenge the professional power of doctors over nurses.

An analysis completed by Touche Ross (DoH and Touche Ross, 1991) identified two main areas of cost benefits:

- identified savings of £15.88 million and £3.45 million per annum in district nursing and health visiting time respectively
- a potential £7.34 million annual saving in GP time.

Community nurses have been prescribing informally for many years and with the introduction of nurse prescribing will now have to accept full responsibility for their decisions (UKCC, 1992). Groves (1999) discussed professional accountability with regard to the issue that not all nurses 'are fully autonomous or hold sufficient power in all aspects of their work to be held to account'. Within nurse prescribing, nurses by law now have the 'power' and autonomy to prescribe from the *Nurse Prescribers' Formulary* (*NPF*), being accountable for the decision-making process from assessment to implementation. Nurse prescribing can be seen to have legitimised the idea of autonomy and enhanced nursing as a profession.

Luker *et al* (1997a) researched the impact within the pilot sites of nurse prescribing in England and how patients perceived the role of nurses. They identified that patients were aware that nurses made many decisions with regard to their treatment and care, but were restricted in its implementation as they needed the GP to sign the prescription. Luker *et al* (1997b) also identified that GPs considered nurses to possess the most appropriate knowledge to prescribe wound care products. Although this was not expanded on in the study, it can be assumed that GPs believe nurses to have more in-depth knowledge of wound healing and product suitability.

Within Ayrshire and Arran Primary Care NHS Trust nurse prescribing was in its second year, at the time of writing, with a total of 127 nurses prescribing. By June 2001 all eligible nurses within the trust will have completed the training necessary to be able to prescribe from the *NPF*. Within the primary care setting in Scotland nurses are now working in Local Health Care Cooperatives (LHCCs), resulting in district nurses and health visitors working more closely with their GP colleagues to meet the needs of the population within the LHCC and individual patients' needs within their GP practice. Nurse prescribing can be seen as enhancing nurses' autonomy and reducing dependence on GP colleagues as nurses are now able to obtain certain drugs and appliances without seeking a GP to sign prescriptions.

By looking at each nurse's prescribing pattern and volume within the Ayrshire and Arran Trust, it can be identified that health visitors prescribe a great deal less than district nurses. This is primarily because of client groups being cared for by health visitors, who deliver health advice and practical support to parents and older people. In 1998–1999, of the provisional 400,000 home visits completed by health visitors nearly half of them were to patients under the age of five years (Scottish Office, 1999). This prescribing pattern has been reflected across the country, as Luker *et al*'s (1988) study shows.

Methodology

The main aim of this research was to examine the issue of nurses' increased autonomy and reduced dependence on GPs in the delivery of patient care since becoming nurse prescribers. The research was also concerned with assessing whether there was an association between years of experience since obtaining the district nursing and/or health visiting qualification and the frequency of prescribing.

As this was a descriptive study, a questionnaire was developed and piloted. The pilot group consisted of nurses with either district nursing or health visiting qualifications who were not prescribing at that time. Ethical approval was discussed, but identified as unnecessary. The rationale for performing a descriptive study was to facilitate the gathering of information in relation to characteristics of individual nurses as well as summarising patterns in the responses of nurses within the sample. This type of study allows for the examination of relationships between different variables, eg. discipline, volume and frequency of prescribing.

Information was collected from questionnaires. The structure of the questionnaire included a combination of open and closed questions. Questions were developed based on the information and variables required in this project. The sequence of questioning was reviewed with the required factual information (eg. qualifications, length of time prescribing) addressed in the first five questions. It was hoped that this would keep the nurse's attention before asking the more detailed open questions that required them to reflect on their practice and beliefs with regard to nurse prescribing. These questions were structured to ensure they were not leading, biased or worded negatively.

The questionnaire was distributed to all nurse prescribers within the trust (n=127). A covering memo was also distributed, highlighting the rationale for the study, with the intention of increasing the return rate of the questionnaires. Completed questionnaires were returned by post, thereby guaranteeing the anonymity of the nurses. The author was the only researcher involved.

Results

Of the 127 questionnaires distributed, ninety were returned completed and legible — a response rate of 71%. Of those who returned the questionnaire, forty-four had district nursing qualifications and forty-six had health visiting qualifications.

Respondents' details

The mean number of years since the nurses had gained their professional qualification was 9.49 years, with a standard deviation of 7.58 years. The range varied from one to thirty years of experience with either a district nursing or health visiting qualification. These numbers do not represent previous years of experience with the nurses' general qualifications.

Since 1998, when nurse prescribing was introduced across the trust, the sample group of nurses had been prescribing for different periods of time and therefore had different levels of experience. In the questionnaire, nurses were asked to identify how long they had been actively nurse prescribing (*Figure 10.1*). Of the eighty-nine nurses who answered this question, thirty-two (36%) had been prescribing for between six months and one year, and forty-seven (53%) for more than one year. The remaining ten (11%) had been prescribing for less than six months.

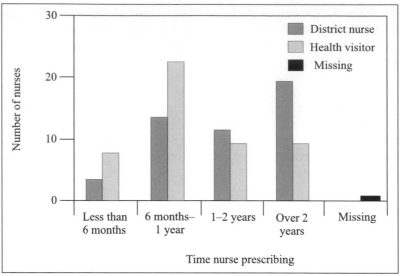

Figure 10.1: Time actively nurse prescribing

Prescribing patterns

The questionnaire asked about the frequency of prescription writing in the month before it was completed. The data were grouped and cross-tabulated with the professional qualifications of the nurses (*Table 10.1*).

For statistical purposes it was assumed that health visitors and district nurses would prescribe at the same frequencies. Therefore, if forty nurse prescribers write less than five prescriptions a month the ratio of district nurses to health visitors in that group would be the same as the overall ratio of district nurses to health visitors in the whole sample (expected count). Divergence of actual counts from the expected counts would indicate that there are differences between district nurse and health visitor prescribing patterns.

The results of the c2 Pearson test suggest a significant relationship between the nurses' qualifications and the frequency of prescription writing, in that district nurses write more prescriptions than health visitors (*Table 10.1*). Fifty-seven per cent of district nurses (n=25) prescribed more than eleven prescriptions in the preceding month, while 70% of health visitors (n=32) indicated that they wrote less than five prescriptions in the same period. This pattern of district nurses prescribing more than health visitors has been previously mentioned and was to be expected.

It could be perceived that nurses who prescribe on a regular basis would be more aware of their dependence on GPs for advice and support; because they are prescribing more frequently, they are more likely to have had the need to access GP advice.

Table 10.1: Cross-tabulation of professional qualifications with prescriptions

Number of prescriptions written in past month		Professional qualifications		
		District nurse	Health visitor	Total
Less than 5	Count	8	32	40
	Expected count	19.6	20.4	40.0
6–10	Count	11	10	21
	Expected count	10.3	10.7	21.0
11–20	Count	14	4	18
	Expected count	8.8	9.2	18.0
Over 20	Count	11	0	11
	Expected count	5.4	5.6	11.0
Total	Count	44	46	90
	Expected count	44.1	45.9	90.0
χ^2 **Pearson** =30.97		3df*	p=0.000	
Minimum expected frequency		= 5.38		
Cells with expected frequency		= <5(0%)		
Cramer's V =0.59				
Missing observations		=0		
*Degrees of freedom				

Views on autonomy and dependence

Of the two key issues being reviewed (autonomy and dependence on GPs), 48% of the ninety nurses who returned the questionnaire agreed with the statement that their autonomy had increased since they became nurse prescribers, 28% strongly agreed, 21% indicated no change in their sense of autonomy and 3% disagreed (*Figure 10.2*). There appears to be no significant difference (p=0.325 two-tailed) between district nursing and health visiting opinion in relation to autonomy.

Of the ninety nurse prescribers, 66.5% (n=55) felt that they had become less dependent on their GP. However, 27% (n=25) felt that there had been no change in the level of their dependence upon GP colleagues, and 3% (3) felt that they had become more dependent on their GP (*Figure 10.3*). Seven of the ninety nurse prescribers did not answer this question.

The two variables (autonomy and dependence) were joined together to give another variable that looked at the overall issue of increased autonomy and reduced dependence. This indicated that overall, 61% (n=55) of the nurses (seven missed observations) either agreed or strongly agreed with both of the questions (*Figure 10.4*). The remaining twenty-eight nurses indicated that they felt there had been no change in their level of autonomy or dependence.

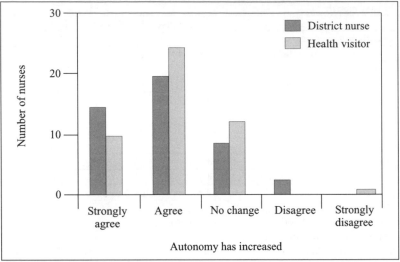

Figure 10.2: Views on level of autonomy

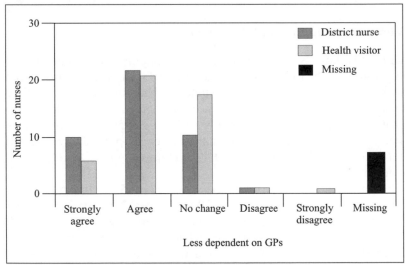

Figure 10.3: Views on level of dependence on GPs

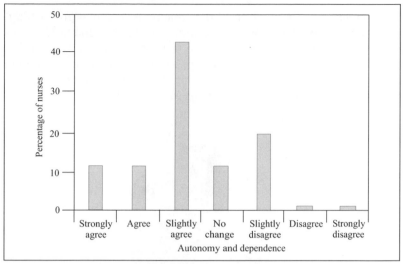

Figure 10.4: Overall picture of increased autonomy and reduced dependence

Using this new variable, the relationship between the perceptions of increased autonomy/reduced dependence and years of experience was tested. Due to the range of years of experience within the sample, this variable was recorded and the years were grouped together into two broad bands: nine years or less and ten years or more. From these data it was found that, in this sample, the relationship between years of experience and opinion on increased autonomy and reduced dependence on GPs is not significant (Mann-Whitney U test p=0.737 two-tailed).

As we have seen, nurses with a district nursing qualification prescribe more frequently than their health visiting colleagues. In this sample there is no significant relationship between professional qualification/volume of prescriptions written and nursing views on autonomy and dependence (p=0.171 two-tailed).

Views on development and GP support

Overall, 90% (n=82) of nurses believed nurse prescribing to be a positive development (eight missing observations) and 80% (n=73) believed that their GPs were supportive of it (thirteen missing observations). In the questionnaire, nurses were asked to quantify their answers to certain questions about their perception on professional development and GPs' reactions to nurse prescribing. The main issues identified are illustrated in the pie charts (*Figures 10.5, 10.6*). All the issues related to the aims of nurse prescribing previously discussed (ie. time saving, additional work being handed over from GPs and challenging the dominance of the medical profession) were identified by nurses in this study.

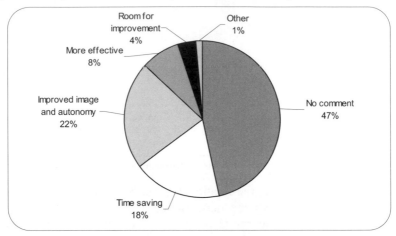

Figure 10.5: Nurse prescribers' views of positive aspects of nurse prescribing

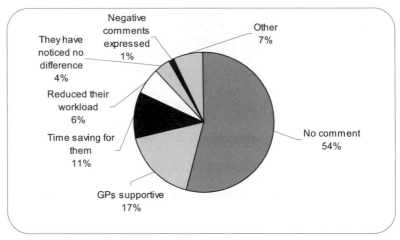

Figure 10.6: Nurse prescribers' views of effect of nurse prescribing on GPs

Forty-eight of ninety nurses expanded on the positive aspects of nurse prescribing. Eighteen per cent of the forty-eight replies identified that it is time saving for the nurse, as they are no longer required to access their GP to write a prescription for an item in the *NPF*, 22% felt that nurse prescribing had improved their image and increased their autonomy as a professional, and 8% commented that they were aware of patient care being delivered in a more effective environment. The nurse is able to write a prescription at the time of assessment, and treatment can commence at that time, rather than at a later date when a prescription written by a GP is acquired. In addition, 4% of the respondents believed that patients could benefit more if the *NPF* was expanded.

Forty-one nurses (46%) expanded on their answers relating to GP support for nurse prescribing. Eleven per cent of the forty-one replies identified that nurse prescribing was saving GPs' time and GPs were supportive of this development, 4% of nurses indicated that their GPs had not noticed any difference and only one nurse stated that the GPs had expressed negative comments.

Limitations and recommendations

It is difficult to ascertain if the results identified in this research would be transferable to other nurse prescribers, as some of the results are based on individuals' perceptions of issues raised. However, it could be imagined that nurse prescribers across the country are faced with many of the same issues. It would have been beneficial, in this study, to ask the nurse prescribers to expand on some of the issues raised in the questionnaire, especially in relation to their perception of autonomy and their present relationship with their GP colleagues. It would be interesting to establish whether there is any effect on autonomy and dependence relating to where nurse prescribers are based, ie. in the surgery/health centre or external accommodation.

Discussion

This study shows that, within this sample, prescribing nurses and their GP colleagues view nurse prescribing as a positive development for the nursing profession. This study has identified that nurses with district nursing qualifications write significantly more prescriptions than their health visitor colleagues. This is related to the client group that the latter visit, namely children under the age of five years and the fact that much of health visitors' work focuses on health promotion among well people. In addition, the majority of items in the original *NPF* are related to wound care, which has been the domain of the client groups visited by district nurses and is recognised as these nurses' area of specialist knowledge.

Although the results indicate that overall, nurses believe their autonomy has increased and their dependence on GPs has reduced, it cannot be demonstrated that there is a significant relationship between the variables, eg. number of prescriptions written, years since obtaining professional qualification and becoming a nurse prescriber. This may be an indication that nurses have been indirectly prescribing for years by asking the GPs for the prescription, but it is only now with the introduction of nurse prescribing that they are receiving the recognition and responsibility for this process.

Conclusion

Nurse prescribing is now a core component of the present training programme necessary to gain either a district nursing or health visiting qualification. With the extension of nurse prescribing now being implemented, to include additional nurses and increase the range of items that can be prescribed, it may be necessary for nurses to seek support and advice from their GPs and community pharmacists. As a trust, we are endeavouring to address this issue by developing an ongoing educational programme to support nurse prescribers, allowing them to retain their autonomy in prescribing by assisting them to remain competent in their prescribing practice.

Key Points

⌘ District nurses tend to prescribe more than health visitors.

⌘ Nurses identified an increase in their autonomy since becoming nurse prescribers as well as a reduction in dependence on GPs.

⌘ There is no relationship between frequency of prescribing and perceptions of autonomy and dependence.

⌘ Nurse prescribing is generally viewed as being a positive development for nursing.

References

Cumberlege J (1986) *Neighbourhood Nursing: A Focus for Care*. HMSO, London

Department of Health and Touche Ross (1991) *Nurse Prescribing Final Report: A Cost Benefit Study*. DoH, London

Groves E (1999) Nurse prescribing — accountability. In: Humphries J, Green J, eds. *Nurse Prescribing*. Palgrave, (formerly Macmillan Press) London/Basingstoke

Luker K, Austin L, Hogg C, Ferguson B, Smith K (1997a) Patients' views of nurse prescribing. *Nurs Times* **93**(17): 51–4

Luker K, Austin L, Hogg C, Ferguson B, Smith K (1997b) Nurses' and GPs' views of the 'Nurse Prescribers' Formulary'. *Nurs Standard* **11**(22): 33–8

Luker K, Austin L, Hogg C, Ferguson B, Smith K (1998) Decision Making: The context of nurse prescribing. *J Adv Nurs* **27**: 657–65

McCartney W, Tyrer S, Brazier M, Prayle D (1999) Nurse prescribing: radicalism or tokenism? *J Adv Nurs* **29**(2): 348–54

National Board for Nursing, Midwifery and Health Visiting for Scotland (1997) *Nurse Prescribing — Open Learning Pack*. NBS, Edinburgh

NHS Executive (1999) *Review of Prescribing, Supply and Administration of Medicines*. NHS Executive, London

Scottish Executive (2001) *Nurses to be Given Wider Prescribing Powers*. News release SE1201/2001. http://www.scotland.gov.uk/news/2001/05/se1201.asp (accessed 22 June 2001)

Scottish Office (1999) *National Health Service in Scotland. Annual Report 1998–99*. http://www.scotland.gov.uk/library2/doc07/nhsar-00.htm (accessed 15 June 2001)

United Kingdom Central Council for Nursing, Midwifery and Health Visiting (1992) *Code of Professional Conduct*. UKCC, London

11

Celebrating the present, challenging the future of nurse prescribing

Lynn Basford, Dianne Bowskill

As universities gear up to deliver the next wave of nurse prescriber training, this chapter — based in part on the experiences of the University of Derby and its partner trusts and the recent consultation document (Department of Health, 2001) and Educational Policy letter (ENB, 2001a) — considers the issues underpinning the education and training of nurse prescribers. The collaborative, cooperative and coordinated approach seen in the training of the first wave facilitated the preparation of large numbers of practitioners to prescribe while maintaining service provision to patients in the community. The success of the programme should be celebrated, but also raises topics for debate as nurse prescribing expands to include a much wider range of nurses. The consultation document identifies the range of medicines from which a new, extended nurse prescribers' formulary has been created and informs the subsequent education policy letter that outlines education and training parameters that will underpin the new prescribing requirements. It is clear that some challenges similar to those experienced during the first wave of nurse prescribing will arise, but there are also some significant differences that have raised pertinent questions and require answers.

The call from government to educate community nurses and health visitors in prescribing has been unique in the history of modern nursing. This phenomenon has challenged not only the prescribing position of medical practitioners but also the isolated and inflexible ways in which educational programmes for nurses work.

Nurse prescribing training programmes necessitated an approach that required educationalists and employers to work collaboratively, effectively, economically and with vision and innovation, and enabled 2002 nurses to be adequately prepared to prescribe competently in a relatively short space of time (English National Board for Nursing,

124

Midwifery and Health Visiting [ENB], 2001a). Juxtaposed with this was the need to maintain, and in some instances enhance or change, the service infrastructure through which care was delivered. It clearly required commitment, organisation, planning and execution at each stage of the process. A model that is necessary to address as curriculum designers prepare programmes for Extended Prescribing. This latest development has been welcomed by the nursing profession and those agents who monitor the quality and effectiveness of patient care that nurse prescribing has achieved. Reflecting on the experience gained it is important that challenges previously presented are learnt and addressed within the new prescribing developments. We will therefore draw on the University of Derby's experiences of the two years in which it has been preparing nurses to prescribe, to offer challenging thoughts for future debates if all health professionals are to share knowledge, skill and understanding of nurse prescribing.

Criteria for success

A major factor for our success was the high degree of collaboration, cooperation and coordination between educationalists, service providers, workforce confederations and health authority leads throughout the project. The process was highly visible and sustained until the last students had achieved independent prescriber status. In achieving and maintaining this level of involvement we adhered to a basic set of principles that chiefly centred on:

- the need to gain and hold mutual respect for one another
- the need to recognise the knowledge and skills each member brought to nurse prescribing.

These two criteria were significant in formulating the basis of our sustained success, in that they enabled us to make effective use of teamworking and networking skills for the benefit of the project. Working to these basic principles enabled the experience, and a common knowledge and understanding of prescribing issues to be shared by everyone. We believe that this outcome was instrumental in achieving the shared goal of enhancing the quality of patient care and educating practitioners to undertake new and demanding roles and responsibilities.

The task of training nurses to prescribe was on a scale never before undertaken in the history of nurse education; from the outset, the planning team drew on their collective wisdom and experience to overcome challenges. These challenges mainly centred on the need to educate large numbers of practitioners in a relatively short time, while maintaining high standards of patient care in the community. We did this primarily by undertaking detailed planning based on workload analysis, followed by some creative thinking to overcome the obstacle of educating the staff concerned and releasing them from their nursing duties.

Our solution was to plan the phased release of staff. A two-year programme timetable was designed and sent to educationalists, managers, and practitioners. This allowed everyone involved to know who was to be released from duties, what cover was needed and where. We then had to design an educational model that offered flexibility while maintaining the constructs of the national education and training guidelines. This flexibility centred on supporting education delivery and taking the final summative examination in the various localities of the trusts.

It was an approach that worked extremely well in supporting ongoing service needs and was instrumental in enabling practitioners who worked in isolated geographical areas to access the programme while feeling individually supported in their locality.

Overall, the educationalists' attitudes and responsiveness towards the delivery of the educational programme received positive accolades from students, service providers and the educational contractors. In addition, the model's flexibility cemented the working relationships between the partner agents and improved collaboration and cooperation beyond contractual obligations. A continuation of development groups set up for the first wave have grown to accommodate the diversity of nurses now able to prescribe particularly in acute sectors. A clear indication that the experience has not been lost and the cooperative venture has been built on for the future education and training of nurse prescribers.

In considering our achievements we are now in a position to celebrate the successful implementation of the first wave of nurse prescribing education and training in our region. However, we are aware that the second wave will be on a different scale and from a much broader legislative base than before, and we acknowledge that there will be different challenges. We believe our experiences with the first wave can be used to inform the debates and the implementation process for new models.

Informing future challenges

The challenges perceived from the many debates and the latest consultation document from the Department of Health (DoH) (2001) suggest that there will still be difficulties in training potential nurse prescribers: the needs of individual practitioners will need to be considered, while simultaneously overcoming the continuing needs of service. However, the document also identifies new issues that require attention from a much wider perspective and will need very different education and training packages. For example, there will be a change in the length of the educational requirement from three taught days to a more comprehensive model of thirty-seven days, which includes developing a knowledge base of a much broader prescribing formulary (ENB/DoH, 2001). There will also be a practical component under the guidance of a medical supervisor who is competent to prescribe (ENB, 2001b).

We believe that these new parameters can only be achieved if key stakeholders have:

- knowledge and understanding of the various issues underpinning prescribing practice
- a willingness and motivation to communicate with others
- the ability to coordinate the education and training with a high degree of cooperation.

We also suggest that there is a fundamental need for flexible models of education and training that are responsive to a wider scope of practitioner and service needs. For example, nurse prescribing practice will no longer be targeted at community nurses who hold either a district nurse or health visitor qualification; it is proposed that a range of specialist nurses will be eligible to undertake prescribing education and training. Eligible nurses may work in fields of practice such as accident and emergency departments, walk-in centres, NHS Direct, palliative care, family planning, chronic disease management and school nursing. This is reflected in the DoH's (2001) consultation document, which extends the *Nurse Prescribers' Formulary* (*NPF*) and increases the opportunities for all first level nurses to be trained to prescribe.

This is intrinsically different to the first prescribing model with its limited scope. The new proposal suggests that first level registered nurses, who have successfully completed an enhanced programme of preparation for nurse prescribing, could prescribe from an extended list that will include a wide range of prescription-only medicines (PoMs). There is no requirement for practical experience which means that nurses could, in theory, proceed straight from registration to the nurse prescribing course, without having consolidated their preregistration education. It can be argued that this is unimportant if they have relevant knowledge, skill, understanding and are competent in their practice. Indeed, the consultation document asserts that under the UKCC's (1992) *Professional Code of Conduct*, their competence should be assured and *The Scope of Professional Practice* (UKCC, 1992) enables nurses to widen their scope, providing they can demonstrate competence.

Nurse prescribing is an exciting challenge for the nursing profession, but there are some issues that require serious consideration. For instance, our experience with specialist community practitioners has shown that not all will be willing or able to take on the new prescribing role. While voluntary access may not seem an obvious issue for debate at the moment, given that extended prescribing requires the practitioner not only to work within any of the four specific therapeutic areas for prescribing but also they are required to assume and maintain competence through practice. The possibility remains that some nurses may find themselves in a prescribing role but may not have the competence or capability to undertake the responsibility and accountability of prescribing.

Competence

Nurse prescribing is an extension of the nurse's role and can be justified under the competence framework. However, the term 'competence' in the DoH's (2001) consultation document is loosely stated and does not account for the depth and range of knowledge, and the level of skill required by the nurse prescriber. However, universities have addressed the standardisation of competence in prescribing through the integration of concepts and competence outcomes identified in 'Maintaining Competency in Prescribing', an outline framework to help nurse prescribers (National Prescribing Centre, 2001). The competency model identified in the document is focused around three domains:

1. The consultation.
2. Prescribing effectively.

3. Prescribing in context.

Each of the three domains has a further three competencies. It is a commonly held view that competence ensures that a practitioner is fit to practice. Fitness for practice assumes that the practitioner has undertaken an appropriate programme of learning with the relevant underpinning knowledge and understanding, and has had experience in practice. Although it could be argued that the first wave of nurse prescribers are 'fit to practice', the changes now occurring mean that they are only competent within a limited scope. This poses questions around their fitness to continue to practice without further education and training. Clearly, the scope of professional practice within the new directives is very different from those identified within the first model. Therefore, those nurses who are qualified as independent nurse prescribers following the previous model are expected to advance clinical knowledge and skills through further education and training (ENB, 2001a). Nurses will need to gain competence in clinical skills that will enable them to make judgements about undifferentiated diagnosis, which means that the patient will not have had their health needs assessed by a doctor or other health professional before visiting the nurse. Nurses will need to learn about physiology, altered physiology, health assessment, diagnostic skills, diagnostic reasoning, pharmacology, the effects of polypharmacy, ethical and legal issues and aspects of clinical governance that reflect their increased accountability and responsibility regarding prescribing. Some consideration to these requirements has been given by the English National Board through the Education Policy letter (2001a) which is indicative of the content for curriculum development.

Voluntary access to education

Education and training to become a nurse prescriber is voluntary and although this respects individual choices to extend the scope of professional practice, there is the potential for disagreement between the employee and the employer. We found that reluctant employees were often strongly recommended to undertake the programme by their employers. This created tension as employees' choices were usurped by peer and employer pressure.

The option not to partake in the extended role of prescribing can be due to a practitioner's closeness to retirement, his/her lack of confidence, or because he/she has limited academic preparation for practice. However, the unwillingness to be a prescriber has significant consequences on the equity of patient care and patients' clarity about who can and cannot prescribe. The latter is particularly significant because attempts are increasingly being made to reduce the gaps between health and social care, thereby somewhat blurring the boundaries between the two.

Patient care needs

The drive for more nurses to prescribe is based on the intention to enhance patient care by providing better continuity of service. The first wave of nurse prescribing training has demonstrated the appropriateness of using nurses to prescribe in the caring setting, using their skills to better effect in the multidisciplinary team (DoH, 2001). However, if nurses choose not to prescribe, their patients and clients will be unlikely to benefit directly from improved continuity of care, creating inequality across the trusts. As effective continuity of service will be reliant on nurses who choose to undertake this role, they will be in greater demand than those who choose not to, particularly in practice areas that are visionary or lack sufficient medical services to fulfil service demands.

Education and training

The DoH's (2001) consultation document recommends that the new training programme for the second wave of nurse prescribers should be extended from three taught days with some time for self-directed study before the examination, to twenty-five taught days and twelve days supervised by a medical practitioner over a three-month period. The programme will remain at level three.

Given the style for the first wave nurse prescribing assessment, the assessment issue is an important one if true competence is to be gauged. The first wave prescribing assessment of competence contained one final examination, which has been criticised. This single summative exam was believed to encourage teaching by didactic instruction and learning by rote. Such approaches limited the opportunities to develop key skills for lifelong learning and to gain skills enabling practitioners to reflect on practice using appropriate evidence. In addition, this style of assessment was not conducive for mature adults to demonstrate their competence, knowledge and skill; rote learning requires a high degree of short-term memory which, psychologists claim, mature adults lose as they grow older (Rogers, 1961). Given that examinations are not conducive to mature students, it is surprising and somewhat disappointing that the extended nurse prescribing model of assessment requires a summative examination. Educationalists have recognised the problem and embraced a seen examination concept that is more conducive to continual professional development and student-centred learning.

The consultation document and requirements for extended prescribing have clearly identified that the practice component is supervised and assessed by a suitably prepared medical practitioner. This has resource implications not only of a financial perspective but also in the replacement of medical practitioner time, and while medical practitioners are willing to devote their time to this activity there are many conflicting constraints, not least patient/client services. There is a positive aspect to what could be seen as an enforced partnership between doctors and nurses in that there is a greater understanding of roles, responsibilities and accountability in health care. In addition, there is greater acknowledged respect for the competence and capability in and between professional groups. It is a model which can be emulated as and when other professional groups become prescribing practitioners breaking down professional barriers, tribalistic behaviours and fragmented care.

Formularies

Since nurses have been able to prescribe there has been much debate by government bodies, nurse leaders, doctors and other health professional groups, to agree on a prescribing formulary. A limited formulary was eventually agreed on for the district nurses and health visitors who had completed the required preparation to become nurse prescribers. Health visitors complained that the list focused too much on the work of district nurses, while district nurses complained it was too limited for them to fulfil their new prescribing role adequately. These statements added weight to the argument to extend the formulary, and were obviously taken into consideration as the second wave of nurse prescribers will be eligible to prescribe from an extended nurses' formulary.

The list of medicines now included in the *NPF* represents those listed in option 3 of the previous consultation document (DoH, 2000a). These include all general sales list (GSL) and pharmacy (P) category medicines and some prescription-only medicines (PoMs). The list of prescription-only medicines has been chosen to reflect the needs of prescribing practitioners working in the following four treatment areas:

- minor ailments
- minor injuries
- health promotion
- palliative care.

The range of medicines includes antibiotics, steroids and analgesics. It is this range that poses a challenge for education providers when promoting shared learning while accommodating the needs of individual groups of nurses in a defined field of practice. This challenge will require curricula that facilitate learning in smaller groups than before, of students who come from diverse specialities and care environments. This may affect the viability of programmes if ways of overcoming such problems are not mapped out in advance. One suggestion is to combine core learning with work-based or distance-learning approaches. This will help maintain a position of shared learning while addressing the needs of practitioners who require a fundamental understanding of the core principles of prescribing and diagnosis, but whose clinical practice will require more depth and scope of knowledge to gain competence in their field. For example, practitioners working in palliative care will focus on the range of palliative medicines and analgesics so that their practice can be enhanced to a high level of competence; while those practitioners working with infectious diseases may focus on having a deeper knowledge and understanding of antibiotics and their various uses.

The extended formulary is a welcome move forward, but poses questions:

❖ Will a two-tier system of nurse prescribers be created and, if so, what will the consequences of this be? In total 20,029 nurses underwent prescribing education and training in the first wave (ENB, 2001a). Their preparation was of shorter duration than this second wave and did not prepare them to prescribe from an extended formulary. With hindsight, this was a flaw in the system that can now be seen to have had a damaging effect on the morale of the individuals concerned. In addition, it will be an economic drain, given that further education and training will be required to bring their knowledge and skills up to the new level. Furthermore, in our experience, not all practitioners will wish to extend their scope of prescribing practice any further.

❖ What are the consequences of continuing professional development for nurses who have undertaken education and training to prescribe, but are not called on to use the full range of their knowledge? What happens when new drugs and treatments supercede the old?

We recognise that the extension to prescribing regulations have identified medical practitioners to be medical supervisors without any formal preparation to assess competencies. This is against all current recommended standards for mentorship by the ENB/DoH (2001) and raises a question relating to ethical and moral issues with respect to:

• standards for preparation of assessors and mentors
• clinical governance.

In 2001, the ENB and DoH produced standards for the preparation of mentors, practice educators and lecturers. While in the first instance it is nursing driven, it is expected that all healthcare professional groups will adhere to the standard requirements. This will encourage the imparting of knowledge and development of skills and the assessment of competence to be a rigorous process that assumes clinical governance is upheld. The agenda for clinical governance is broad and diverse, but in the framework of prescribing practice we hope potential and actual problems will be avoided, given that we now know how the continuation of mode 2 is integrated within the specialist programmes of preparation for district nurses and health visitors. There remains however a potential problem as practitioners educated and trained within different models will not be discernable in clinical practice, serving to confuse not only the public and patients but also professionals. The extension of nurse prescribing has created two levels of prescribing in clinical practice, the problems of which are likely to be compounded as we move towards supplementary prescribing creating a third level.

If the parameters for prescribing continue to change, do we continue adopting new education and training programmes for all prescribers or, with a longer-term vision, will practitioners have the inherent skills to seek out new evidence for practice? In our opinion, this should be a mandatory requirement under the auspices of clinical governance and would satisfy the idea that nurse prescribing practitioners have the skills to advance their practice through continual professional development and the notion of lifelong learning.

These questions do not have easy answers, but if the nursing profession is to engage in these developing roles, solutions need to be agreed and acted on by the government, nurse leaders and members of other professional groups. It is clear that there will always be a need for nurse prescribers, particularly given the potential shortage of GPs and the subsequent need to reform health and social care. Professional roles and responsibilities should be extended beyond the boundaries that are, at the very best, artificial in the caring environment. For example, patient care needs do not discretely fit in either the health or social domain, but may cross the two. This demands that health and social care practitioners work collaboratively and cooperatively to provide the best possible care.

Conclusion

Educating and training nurses to prescribe has been a challenging and rewarding experience. The collective body of knowledge and skills gained in undertaking this project over the two-year period has allowed us to inform current debates and challenge some of the issues emerging in the new consultation document and general discourse. The direction put forward in *The NHS Plan* (DoH, 2000b) suggests that nurses will take on more leading roles that extend their current scope of professional practice. Nurse prescribing is here to stay, however, its nature and application will change over time with further experience and professional maturity. The changing nature of nurse prescribing needs a more visionary perspective and collaborative policy direction to provide a clear and comprehensive framework to support nurses in prescribing, and to advance their knowledge and skill within the constructs and boundaries of professional and legal accountability.

In this chapter, we have used our experiences to raise issues that need to be resolved. We believe that education should be flexible and clinically-based to achieve competence. In addition, it should encourage the development of skills that foster lifelong learning and the seeking of evidence of best practice.

Nurse prescribing is in its infancy; historians will look back on this period of time and comment on the process and outcome of the new development. We should build on the foundation developed so far and ensure that the next generation of nurse prescribers will be fit for purpose and for practice. Being part of this collaborative venture will mean that we can celebrate our experiences while trying to overcome the challenges of the future.

Key Points

⌘ Successful implementation of the first wave of nurse prescribers required collaboration, cooperation and coordination.

⌘ The primary intention of proposals to extend nurse prescribing is the enhancement of patient care.

⌘ The Education policy letter, ENB (2001) sets a greater length and depth of education preparation for extended nurse prescribers.

⌘ Issues surrounding assessment, competence and the preparation of medical supervisors require resolution.

⌘ The educational preparation of existing nurse prescribers should be considered in the light of new education proposals.

References

Department of Health (2000a) *Consultation on Proposals to Extend Nurse Prescribing.* October 25th, DoH, London

Department of Health (2000b) *The NHS Plan.* DoH, London

Department of Health (2001) *Extended Prescribing of Prescription Only Medicines By Independent Nurse Prescribers.* MLX 273. 19th July, DoH, London

English National Board/Department of Health (2001) *Preparation for Mentors and Teachers: A Framework of Guidance.* ENB, London

English National Board (2001a) *Education Policy Letter 2001/01/TL September.* ENB, London

English National Board (2001b) *Building on Success.* Annual report 2000–2001 Table 37. ENB, London

National Prescribing Centre (2001) *Maintaining Competency in Prescribing. An outline framework to help nurse prescribers.* NPC, Liverpool

Rogers RC (1961) *A Therapist's View of Psychotherapy: On Becoming a Person.* Constable, London

United Kingdom Central Council for Nursing, Midwifery and Health Visiting (1992) *Code of Professional Conduct.* UKCC, London

United Kingdom Central Council for Nursing, Midwifery and Health Visiting (1992) *Scope of Professional Practice.* UKCC, London

12

Community nurses' contribution to oral health

Jenny Gallagher, Jean Rowe

Oral health is an important component of general health and well-being. Although oral health has improved dramatically in children and young adults, oral diseases remain common, particularly among disadvantaged and vulnerable groups. Many patients seen by community nurses will fall into these categories and are less likely to have sought treatment. This chapter presents the epidemiology of oral diseases and conditions for specific groups in society that community nurses will be caring for. It looks at prescribing principles and describes treatment and advice for common oral conditions, including those where prescription may be appropriate. Community nurses play an important role in the oral health care of society, particularly among those least likely to access dental services.

Community nurses may make a valuable contribution to the oral health of individuals and communities. This chapter provides an overview of the epidemiology of common diseases and conditions which impact on oral health for key client groups: infants and mothers, older people and vulnerable people with special needs who might come under the care of one or more groups of community nurses. It outlines an approach for patient assessment, taking into account oral health issues and their management, setting prescribing within the overall contribution to oral health for these groups.

The ability to prescribe currently recognises the autonomy of appropriately qualified district nurses and health visitors (and some practice nurses with either of these qualifications) where they may be able, through assessment, to offer quick, time-saving and effective treatment. One of the principle advantages of nurse prescribing is that prescriptions can be written in the home, or advice on over-the-counter (OTC) preparations provided, thereby reducing the need for visits to the doctor's or dentist's surgery, especially for people who are house-bound and those with additional social challenges (Humphries and Green, 1999). However, because prescribable oral care items are few, nurse prescribers' clinical contribution is essentially in the wider sphere of promoting oral health through timely advice on diet, cleaning and the purchase of OTC products to support oral health, as well as facilitating access to dental care (Health Education Authority [HEA], 1996a, b).

It is important to recognise that the impact of oral conditions on an individual's life can be profound (Locker, 1992) and good oral health can contribute to individuals' general health and well-being (Fiske *et al*, 2000). Client groups such as adults with learning disabilities have requested greater support in accessing dental care (Pratelli, 2000) and community nurses can play an important role in liaising with the appropriate member of the local dental community for an appointment or domiciliary visit (Bentley *et al*, 1993; HEA, 1996a; Gallagher, 1998; British Society for Disability and Oral Health [BSDH] *et al*, 2001). The following sections describe epidemiological trends in oral diseases and conditions, and uptake of NHS dental services, taking key client groups in turn.

Infants

In infants, oral infection with the yeast Candida albicans (oral thrush or candidosis) may interfere with breastfeeding. Scully and Cawson (1998) suggested that thrush is common in the newborn, in whom it may resolve spontaneously or in response to antifungal treatment. It is one type of oral candidosis, producing soft creamy-white patches that can be wiped off the soft tissues of the mouth leaving red areas, particularly on the palate and cheeks. Treatment is required where the mother experiences pain on breastfeeding and there is visual evidence of oral thrush in the infant. Mothers may require support to continue breastfeeding during this potentially difficult period.

Traditionally, antifungal medication is prescribed for the infant in the form of nystatin oral suspension. The suspension is placed by dropper in the child's mouth just before breastfeeding, so treating the infant and mother simultaneously (Booth, 1994; HEA, 1998). There is little published evidence on the prevalence of oral thrush in infants and the effectiveness of this intervention; however a small study of thirty-five infants by Boon *et al* (1989) suggested that ketaconazole was more successful than nystatin in curing oral thrush in infants. A larger German study reported by Hoppe (1997) showed that miconazole gel was significantly superior to nystatin suspension in achieving cure. By day 12 of treatment, 97% of the miconazole group were cured compared with 54% of the nystatin group. However, there are contraindications to the use of miconazole and the *Nurse Prescribers' Formulary* (*NPF*) advises caution in the case of breastfeeding. Further trials on its use may be advised and nystatin considered a more acceptable first line of treatment.

Tooth eruption (ie. 'teething') may also cause problems, although prevalence of teething problems is a subject of discussion among dentists and paediatricians. Tooth eruption is a slow process, taking on average two months (Hulland *et al*, 2000). Two recent prospective studies of infants reported in a series of papers (Hulland *et al*, 2000; Macknin *et al*, 2000; Wake *et al*, 2000) have found no conclusive evidence that a consistent relationship exists between the eruption of teeth and the experience of symptoms such as fever, dribbling, flushed cheeks, rashes, diarrhoea etc. One of the studies (Hulland *et al*, 2000) did report that the appearance in the mouth of baby teeth is commonly, but not consistently, accompanied by redness of the gingival tissues. Although there was no clear pattern, the researchers could not rule out the possibility that weak associations may exist. Research findings to date therefore contrast with centuries of strong beliefs to the contrary (Ashley, 2001) but, if valid, Wake *et al* suggest that they need to be taken seriously to ensure that common patterns of illness and behaviour in young children are appropriately managed. In light of the above findings, Frank and Drezner (2001) recommend that temperature greater than 38°C and other serious symptoms should be evaluated appropriately and not automatically be attributed to teething.

It is not surprising, considering the problems in diagnosing teething, that there is no firm evidence-base for its treatment. Current best practice includes cold teething rings, teething gels which are available OTC or prescription of paracetamol suspension (Steward, 1988; HEA, 1996a). There are several lidocaine-based gels available, homeopathic powders and a choline salicylate gel. The latter is not recommended for very young children. In light of the above findings it would seem appropriate that these are merely short-term measures, prior to seeking medical advice. This is an area requiring further research and the development of evidence-based guidelines.

The early weaning period provides opportunities for oral health promotion, which could influence good dental health behaviour in the family. Key messages for dental health promotion in children include:

❖ Diet: reduce intake of sugary food and drink.

❖ Tooth-brushing: clean teeth thoroughly twice every day with a pea-sized amount of fluoride toothpaste from when the teeth first erupt.

❖ Dental attendance: encourage regular dental visits from an early age (Chestnutt *et al*, 1998).

Changing oral health behaviour is a complex process (Kent and Croucher, 1998). Dental attendance for an oral examination is recommended at least once per year although there is no evidence to support one fixed recall interval for all individuals, particularly in light of changing disease patterns. The Scientific Basis of Dental Health Education (HEA, 1996b) recommended that people seek an oral examination every year, but that children and people determined to be at high risk may need to be seen more frequently. As well as treating oral disease, dental professionals may provide specific oral health promotion. In a review of current evidence Kay and Locker (1997) concluded that interventions in the dental surgery aimed at improving oral hygiene were effective.

Children

Although national and local surveys have revealed vast improvement in the levels of tooth decay over the past few decades (*Figure 12.1*) (O'Brien 1994; Downer, 1998), children are still more at risk of developing tooth decay than any other oral condition. By the age of five years, 40% of children have experienced tooth decay and have, on average, four decayed teeth (Pitts *et al*, 2001). This rises to approximately 60% of fifteen-year olds (O'Brien, 1994).

Clear inequalities in oral health exist. Although there has been a reduction in the average levels of disease, many surveys have demonstrated the association between oral health and social deprivation at all ages (O'Brien, 1994; Hinds and Gregory, 1995; Pitts, 1998; Sweeney *et al*, 1999), with children from lower social classes experiencing higher levels of decay (*Figure 12.2*). A national diet and nutrition survey of pre-school children showed that social and educational status were more closely associated with dental caries than dietary history such as sugar intake (Hinds and Gregory, 1995).

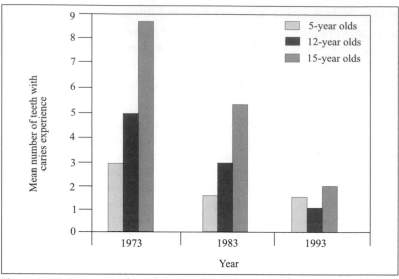

Figure 12.1: Mean number of decayed, missing and filled teeth in children in England and Wales by age, 1973–1993 (from O'Brien, 1994)

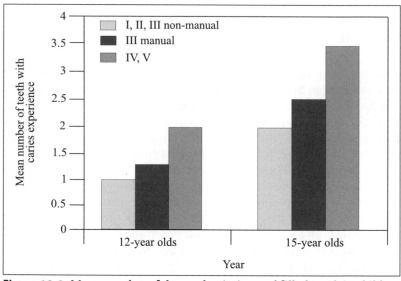

Figure 12.2: Mean number of decayed, missing and filled teeth in children in England and Wales by age and social class, 1973–1993 (from O'Brien, 1994)

Maguire (1996) showed that chronically-sick children (eg. those with epilepsy, cystic fibrosis, chronic renal failure, asthma) who took long-term liquid oral medicines had significantly more caries of deciduous anterior teeth than their healthy siblings. It seems likely that many of the same children who require support from health visitors and community nurses because of medical and social issues are at higher risk of developing or having untreated oral disease.

Durward and Thou (1997) recommended that where prescribed or OTC medicines do contain sugar, their caries effect should be minimised where possible by taking the medication in tablet form; brushing with a fluoride toothpaste or chewing sugar-free gum after taking the medicine; taking medicines at mealtimes; and avoiding ingestion of medicine before going to bed. However, increased availability and use of sugar-free liquid medicines is of course preferable (Mackie and Bentley, 1994; Durward and Thou, 1997).

Young children are the least likely age group to visit a dentist (*Figure 12.3*) and dental attendance levels are worse in areas of social deprivation such as inner-London (Dental Practice Board [DPB], 2001). Innovative community schemes which are 'more than a one-off initiative' have the potential to promote good oral health as part of general healthy living in a supportive environment where health professions are working collaboratively on a 'common risk factor approach' (Sprod *et al*, 1996) such as Sure Start (Department for Education and Employment/Department of Health [DoH], 2000). Many health visitors may currently be working on the 'Brushing for Life Campaign' providing regular toothpaste and brushes for infants and their siblings in areas of high disease over the next three years (Secretary of State for Health, 2000; DoH, 2001c).

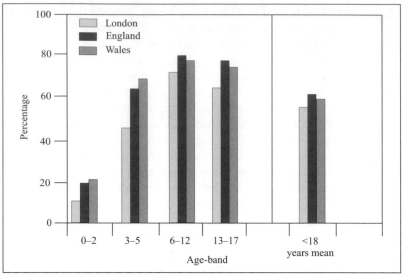

Figure 12.3: Registration under GDS: children (from Dental Practice Board, 2001). London is the worst health region in the country with regards to child dental health

Young adults

Young adults (16–24 years) in the UK now have little experience of tooth decay (Kelly *et al*, 2000). They also may have little experience of accessing dental services, or awareness of their need to do so, yet they remain at risk of dental disease. Kelly *et al*'s national survey (2000) revealed that they have the most untreated decay of all adult age groups. The same study showed that people in the sixteen to twenty-four age group have not increased their dental attendance patterns in line with the rest of the adult population. Almost half (48%) of these young adults nationally said that they attended a dentist less often than they did five years previously (Kelly *et al*, 2000; Nuttal *et al*, 2001).

Young adults become independent and have to develop their own health-related behaviours as they move into adulthood (Nuttal *et al*, 2001). Dental attendance requires triggers (Kent and Croucher, 1998); events such as parenthood may trigger dental attendance and this could be encouraged by community nurses — especially health visitors — with responsibilities for supporting expectant and nursing mothers for whom NHS dental care remains free.

Older people

Nationally there are clear trends in the oral health and service use of older people. Older people are now much less likely to have lost all their teeth and wear complete dentures (Kelly *et al*, 2000). However complete dentures are still very common, particularly among older adults who may have lost their natural teeth many years ago, and a decreasing but significant proportion of the population will wear complete or part dentures for the foreseeable future (Kelly *et al*, 2000; Steele *et al*, 2000). For some adults who do have all of their teeth removed, the emotional effects of tooth loss can be profound, even if they are apparently coping well with their dentures. These effects include a sense of bereavement, lowered self-confidence, altered self-image and dislike of appearance, an inability to discuss this taboo subject or altered behaviour in socialisation and forming close relationships (Fiske *et al*, 1998). It could be helpful for health professionals providing support for clients making the transition to complete dentures to be aware of the complexity of this transition. Fiske *et al* recommended careful preparation for tooth loss by the dental profession, but perhaps it is district or community nurses — who are in regular contact with a client — who may spot these signs in a patient whom 'the dentist' considers is coping with dentures.

Older people who retain their teeth present different challenges to health professionals. They remain at risk of tooth decay — in fact their risk of decay increases as they age — and gum recession leads to exposed dentine root surfaces, which are particularly susceptible to root caries (Steele *et al*, 1998). This happens at a time when manual dexterity and oral hygiene may be declining and diet may be unfavourably high in sugar (Steele *et al*, 1998). One easy measure for older people to take to try to reduce tooth decay is to ensure that they use high-strength fluoride toothpaste (1500ppm) which will provide greatest protection against caries (Holt and Murray 1997). Many (though not all) commercially produced toothpastes contain this concentration of fluoride.

In general, adults over seventy-five years of age are less likely to seek dental care regularly than the rest of the adult population (Dental Practice Board [DPB], 2001). In England, registration for dental care stands at 45% for adults (*Figure 12.4*). This low level could be because patients are only registered for a fifteen-month period with their dentist, as opposed to permanently with their doctor. Problems can arise when patients think that they have a 'relationship' with a dentist only to find that their NHS registration has lapsed and their dentist may no longer be willing to accept new registrations or re-registration because of a shift towards the private sector. Over 25% of primary dental care is now considered to be provided privately, although only 6% of dental practices offer exclusively private care (British Dental Association, 2000). This will vary from place to place depending on dentists' philosophies and local economies, but it is unlikely that private care uptake will be high for this population group, many of whom will be living on low income and experiencing other life challenges such as poor health and impaired mobility. In areas such as London, the uptake of dental care by older people is particularly low (*Figure 12.4*). Another important point to note is that older people are not automatically exempt from charges and will have to pay the necessary 80% of costs up to a level of £360.00 (as of 1 April 2001) unless they are on income support.

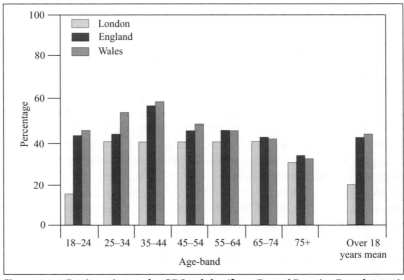

Figure 12.4: Registration under GDS: adults (from Dental Practice Board, 2001)

The incidence of oral cancer increases with age, with 85% of cases in the UK occurring in people aged fifty years or over (Cancer Research Campaign [CRC], 2000). In the UK there are approximately 3500 new cases each year in total (CRC, 2000). The initial symptoms include an ulcer/sore which fails to heal or bleeds easily, a white/red patch that will not go away, a lump or thickening of the oral tissues in the mouth, throat or on the tongue, difficulty in chewing or swallowing, or new persistent pain (CRC, 2000). Clients may present late for care as the early stages are asymptomatic. The most important risk factors are smoking and alcohol consumption (particularly together) and the chewing of betel nut with tobacco (Johnson, 1991). There is some evidence of higher incidence of oral cancer among people of Asian origin (Warnakulasuriya *et al*, 1999). Smoking/tobacco cessation programmes will contribute to good oral and general health.

People with specific needs

Community nurses may see a higher proportion of people with specific needs than the vast majority of the dental profession. Although it is not possible to examine all of these groups in this chapter, three of those with the greatest likelihood of oral problems are:

* patients with cancer
* HIV+ patients
* patients with learning difficulties.

Patients with cancer

It is very important that the oral and medical care of cancer patients are integrated, particularly for patients with any lesions requiring radiotherapy in the head and neck area. Radiotherapy damages the salivary glands, causing dry mouth and increasing the risk of dental disease (Scully and Cawson, 1998). The oral health of patients should be assessed formally and all dental conditions should be treated before radiotherapy is commenced. Oral complications are common among patients with advanced cancer (Sweeney and Bagg, 2000). Patients may experience problems with oral hygiene procedures, pain, oral infections and xerostomia (dry mouth) which affect their quality of life. Oral care can contribute to the general well-being of patients with cancer of the head and neck, therefore, alleviation of pain and prevention of infection in the oral cavity should be a priority in providing total, active comfort for the patient (Paunovich *et al*, 2000). Nurses' links with patients will often be precisely because of their underlying condition, but occasionally oral symptoms such as candidal infection may herald new pathology or a degeneration of a patient's condition. Referral to a specialist team may well be indicated and should be undertaken as swiftly as possible (Scully and Cawson, 1998).

Patients with HIV

Many patients with HIV will be attending one or more specialists for care and it is helpful to have a full picture of their health profile, as liaison via the GP or general dental practitioner (GDP) may be more appropriate than community nurse intervention. Patients with HIV infection need regular dental care and good oral hygiene to avoid HIV periodonal disease (Greenspan and Greenspan, 1991). Oral manisfestations of HIV infection include candidiasis, hairy leuko-plakia, specific forms of periodontal disease, Kaposi's sarcoma and non-Hodgkin's lymphoma (EC & WHO, 1993). Ulcers in people with HIV may be a sign of systemic disease. These patients also have a high incidence of herpes infections. Candidal infection may occur following a course of antibiotics or due to poor dental hygiene, but the causes may be much more complex and require specialist expertise. Candida is present in all mouths. It is both a commensal and an oral pathogen (Scully *et al*, 1994) and only causes problems such as oral thrush in infants or when there has been an upset to the oral flora, or in medically compromised children and adults (Scully *et al*, 1994; Scully and Cawson, 1998). Its significance as a 'disease of the diseased' was recognised again with the advent of HIV and AIDS (Scully and Cawson, 1998). Nurse prescribers should not rush in to prescribe for such conditions unless it is part of an agreed package of care, particularly as new treatment regimes are being used which are more than merely the prescription of nystatin pastilles (Scully *et al*, 1994; Eyeson *et al*, 2000).

Candidosis is just one of a range of oral mucosal and periodontal lesions associated with HIV infection and disease progression; these are often symptomatic and require treatment as well as having a diagnostic and prognostic role in the management of the underlying HIV disease (Eyeson *et al*, 2000). Regular oral examinations are therefore very important for people with HIV. Children with specific needs, such as those with HIV infection or those on long-term medication (who may have been receiving medicine in sugar-based formulations), should be considered at high risk of caries and receive supportive dental care that includes the use of sugar-free medicines where possible (Eldridge and Gallagher, 2000).

Patients with learning difficulties

Adults with learning difficulties are increasingly living in the community (BSDH, 2001). However, a survey of adults from a disability case register in one English health authority showed that community-living adults were significantly more likely to have untreated decay than those in institutions (Tiller *et al*, 2001). Such adults living in the community have greater levels of tooth decay than their residential counterparts, and are less likely to access dental services regularly. Tiller *et al* found that poor oral hygiene was common in both groups. Although such adults are autonomous individuals, it is important that health professionals take care to ensure that their dental needs are met (BSDH *et al*, 2001).

Not all groups of people with specific needs are at greater risk of oral and dental disease (BSDH *et al*, 2001). However, for many the challenges of accessing and receiving dental care may be great, even life-threatening, hence the need for a preventive approach to oral disease.

Assessment of clients' health including oral conditions

The philosophy behind the introduction of nurse prescribing is that the practitioner who assesses and diagnoses a medical condition should be responsible for prescribing the treatment (Campbell and Collins, 2001). Community nurses have the clinical skills and expertise to assess and diagnose many problems that they commonly experience with clients and patients (Humphries and Green, 1999), including wide ranging factors that might affect oral health (DoH, 2001a). Health visitors and district nurses are likely to assess pregnant women, mothers with children, older people and other clients with specific medical or social needs. It is worth remembering that senior dentists in the local community dental service or personal dental service may be seeing much the same client group. They remain therefore useful contacts when an urgent opinion is needed or a domiciliary visit is required for a patient who does not have a regular dentist of his/her own (Gallagher, 1998).

The introduction of nurse prescribing for district nurses and health visitors has made them more accountable for their actions. Therefore, a health assessment must include wide-ranging factors that might affect oral health. Oral health assessment procedures could be incorporated into a general health assessment and require information regarding current and past symptoms as well as medical, dental and social histories (*Box 12.1*). Community nurses should be able to access advice and information from their dental or medical colleagues — particularly if there is a predisposing medical condition — or facilitate access to primary care colleagues should this be advocated, based on the assessment.

Box 12.1: Ten steps to oral assessment and care

1. Clarify symptoms: length, severity, treatments etc.
2. Medical history: conditions, drugs, smoking, alcohol etc.
3. Dental history: attendance, treatment, recurrent problems etc.
4. Social history: family support, benefits, diet, oral hygiene etc.
5. Oral assessments includes:

   ❖ lips: colour, moisture, lesions
   ❖ soft tissue: colour, texture, lesions
   ❖ saliva: too much, too little
   ❖ tongue: colour and texture, lesions
   ❖ teeth: fillings, cavities, sharp edges, debris present
   ❖ dentures: present or absent, relationship to any lesion
   ❖ gums: colour, shape, evidence of bleeding, evidence of teeth appearing.
6. Diagnosis.
7. Advice and/or treatment.
8. Referral for care within primary care team.
9. Keep good health records.
10. Review, reassess and support.

Whatever treatment or advice is offered, patients/clients will need information and explanations about it. The shared decision making or concordance needs to be accompanied by explanation of what the prescription is for, how long it might take to work, how it should be taken or used and what action to take if there are side-effects (Royal Pharmaceutical Society of Great Britain, 1997). For some patients, affordability may be an issue, especially for families on a low income and those who cannot access benefits. This is where good advice and information on the most reasonable treatment needs to be assessed against the risk of not doing anything at all (*Box 12.2*). The cost of a prescription may be more than the cost of buying the product OTC, but for those who are exempt from prescription charges, issuing a prescription would be the best option. It is often necessary to give advice on OTC prescriptions, eg. sugar-free paracetamol for children with diabetes and medically-compromised children on long-term medication who should avoid sugar-based medications for the sake of their general and oral health (HEA, 1996a, b; Maguire *et al*, 1996). Community nurses still have the responsibility of assessing and advising patients even though they may wish to buy OTC medication. Pharmacists have particular expertise in these cases and as they are more familiar with current products on the market, clients should be encouraged to contact them.

Box 12.2: Principles of good prescribing

❖ Assess holistic needs of the client: is a prescription necessary?
❖ Consider an appropriate strategy
❖ Consider choice of product
❖ Negotiate contract and achieve concordance with the patient
❖ Review the patient on a regular basis
❖ Ensure record keeping is both accurate and up-to-date
❖ Reflect on prescribing

Source: National Prescribing Centre, 1999

When care has been advised, including the giving of prescriptions, reassessment and follow-up should also be offered. Review is necessary to establish whether the treatment has been effective, safe and acceptable. Acceptability is part of concordance and if medication neither suits the patient nor is easy to administer, further consideration needs to be given with regard to treatment. Most importantly, all key findings and actions taken should be recorded in patient notes and parent-held records. In addition, a record needs to be made in the GP notes to guarantee that this information is shared between all practitioners and carers.

Prescribable drugs

The disadvantage of the *NPF* at present, is that it comprises a relatively limited list of products. However the list may be extended to include drugs such as antibiotics (DoH, 2001b), products that nurses are very familiar with and for which they have had to request GPs to prescribe. The current list of prescribable drugs for patients with oral conditions is contained in *Table 12.1*, together with OTC preparations and suggested actions, although it should be noted that it is not possible to cover every eventuality.

Table 12.1: Assessment of common oral conditions for nurse prescribers (Preparations and drugs in bold are those currently prescribable by qualified nurse prescribers)

Conditions	Common symptoms	Visual examination	Other information	Advice and treatment	Referral	Follow-up
		Assessment		Action		
Teething	Possibly distress Mild pyrexia Excess saliva Tendency to chew on objects No other illness	Slight redness of gums, evidence of tooth erupting	Baby teeth generally appear 6–30 months And adult teeth from 5–6 years	**Paracetamol oral suspension** for 24 hours **Lignocaine-based teething gels** Keep mouth clean	If persists see GP in case other cause of ill health	Ensure symptoms resolve Time for oral hygiene instruction: brush with thin smear of fluoride paste
Dental pain due to toothache or dental abscess	Sensitive to hot and cold stimuli Constant throbbing pain	May be evidence of tooth decay but a filling may obscure any evidence of decay	Dental history	Urgent dental attendance Suitable **analgesia**, eg. **paracetamol** or **aspirin** if delay in dental appointment	General dental practitioner or local emergency dental service or use NHS direct	Encourage dental attendance to complete care Supportive dietary and hygiene advice Use fluoride toothpaste
Gum infection	Bad taste in mouth Dull pain Swollen gums Bleeding on brushing	Red and swollen gums: widespread or localised	Tooth cleaning history — people often stop cleaning when gums are bleeding or painful	Good oral hygiene Limited use of **analgesics** if required as interim measure Chlorhexidine (Corsodyl) mouthwash	Seek dental care including professional cleaning and oral hygiene instruction	Support oral health care regimen advised — note behaviour change is not easy
Dry mouth	Often associated with radiotherapy to head and neck, salivary gland disease or drug interactions Difficulty in eating biscuits Takes constant sips of water	Reduced saliva Sticky or frothy saliva Lack of pooling of saliva in the floor of the mouth	Check if patient is sucking sugary sweets — these will lead rapidly to tooth decay if the client has natural teeth. Check patient's medication	Determine if cause can be eliminated Consider prescribing **Thymol/Glycerin** mouthwash (interim). Ensure that patient receives regular dental care	Liaise with GP if due to medication Liaise with GP or GDP for referral to specialist if persistent underlying cause	If have natural teeth, clients need support to prevent tooth decay — avoidance of frequent sugary intake, good oral hygiene, saliva substitutes etc including plain water

Table 12.1: cont.

Mouth ulcers	Painful ulcer or painless ulcer	Check if single or multiple, recurrent or first such episode. Is it associated with edge of a denture or sharp tooth? Risk factors for oral cancer include tobacco and alcohol (especially together)	Beware of a painless ulcer or an ulcer which persists for more than 3 weeks as this may be evidence of malignancy. If there is general malaise then the ulcers may be viral. If recurrent then apthous stomatitis	Leave dentures out as much as possible. Advise on use of OTC medications, eg. **corsodyl mouth-wash** or **orabase ointment** Limited use of **analgesics**, eg. paracetamol, particularly if viral infection	Assist with dental appointment, particularly if there are concerns about possible malignancy	Ensure that the mouth ulcer has resolved completely and underlying condition (eg. denture) has been dealt with
Candida (thrush) in baby	Mother experiencing pain on breastfeeding	Baby has typical oral candida lesions		**Nystatin oral suspension**		Support mother to continue breast-feeding
Candida (thrush) in child or adult	Pain under top denture or painful soft tissues in immunocompromised patient. Extensive white patches	Red patch under denture or white patch on soft tissues which, when rubbed off, leaves red bleeding	May be associated with recent antibiotic or found in an already immunocompromised patient, eg. post radiotherapy or use of inhalers	Good denture hygiene (if appropriate) Consider **Nystatin pastilles** if no other underlying concerns or treatment approved by specialist. Wash out mouth after inhalers (if used)	Liaison with GP or GDP especially if underlying condition to ensure that you support appropriate care for this client and they seek specialist advice if necessary. Check diabetes if no other known cause	Support good oral hygiene and dental care. Support client in dealing with underlying condition
Cracked lips	Painful cracked lips	Possibly fissured	If denture-wearer, may need new centures	**Paraffin wax** Miconazole gel to lips and mouth	Seek dental check-up if persists	Support dental attendance if required
Bad breath	Patient or others complain of bad breath	May be evidence of poor oral hygiene and debris	Usually poor oral hygiene and infection in mouth	Improve oral hygiene Chlorhexidine (Corsodyl) mouth-wash	Seek dental check-up if it does not resolve	Support good oral hygiene and dental care
Furred tongue	Furred, hairy or coated tongue	Thick coating on tongue which may even be black and 'hairy'	Poor oral hygiene Smoking	Clean tongue with toothbrush or scraper Reduce smoking	Seek dental check-up if it does not resolve	Support good oral hygiene

Conclusion

Good oral health, can make a major contribution to the well-being of individuals. Community nurses have an important role to play through innovative health promotion initiatives at the population level and, in the care of individual clients, through consideration of their oral health status. This will involve providing timely advice, support, referral and, if appropriate, prescription for patients, following full assessment and appropriate liaison with other members of the primary care team. The expanded role of many community nurses to include prescribing means that oral health assessment is an even more important part of general assessment. Therefore, a deeper understanding of oral conditions and their management is vital.

Acknowledgement

Dr JM Zakrzewska, Senior Lecturer/Hon Consultant in Oral Medicine, St Bartholomew's and the Royal London School of Dentistry, Queen Mary, London

Key Points

❋ Tooth decay and gum disease are the most common oral conditions.

❋ Community nurses play an important role in promoting good oral health and facilitating access to dental care at population level and with individual clients.

❋ Vulnerable groups may require additional support in a community setting to achieve good oral health.

❋ Oral conditions may be more common in client groups seen by community nurses.

❋ Senior dentists in the local community dental service may see much the same client groups as community nurses and are therefore useful contacts when either an urgent opinion or a domiciliary visit for a patient who does not have a regular dentist of their own is needed.

References

Ashley MP (2001) It's only teething… a report of the myths and modern approaches to teething. *Br Dent J* **191**: 4–8

Bentley EM, Holloway PJ (1993) An evaluation of the role of health visitors in encouraging infant dental attendance. *Community Dent Health* **10**(3): 243–9

Booth B (ed) (1994) *Over the Counter Formulary: an Authoritative Guide to Preparations Available Without Prescription.* Nursing Times Publication/Macmillan Publications, Basingstoke: 9

Boon JM, Lafeber HN, Mannetje AH, van Olphen AH, Smeets HL, Toorman J, van der Vlist GJ (1989) Comparison of ketoconazole suspension and nystatin in the treatment of newborns and infants with oral candidosis. *Mycoses* **32**(6): 312–15

British Dental Association (2000) *NHS/Private Split. British Dental Association Quarterly Bulletin.* British Dental Association, London: October

British Society for Disability and Oral Health, Faculty of Dental Surgery Diana Princess of Wales Memorial Fund (2001) *Clinical guidelines and integrated care pathways for the oral health care of people with learning disabilities.* Faculty of Dental Surgery, London

Campbell P, Collins G (2001) Prescribing for community nurses. *Nurs Times* **97**(28): 38–9

Chestnutt I, Taylor M, McLay L (1998) Promoting oral health: the role of the health visitor. *Community Practitioner* **71**: 7–8

Cancer Research Campaign (2000) *CRC Cancer Stats: Oral – UK.* Cancer Research Campaign, London

Dental Practice Board (2001) *DPB Registrations: GDS Quarterly Statistics, January–March 2001.* Dental Data Services, Eastbourne

DfEE/DoH (2000) *Sure Start: Making a difference for children and families.* DfEE Publications, Nottingham

Department of Health (1989) *Health Services Management: The Future Development of the Community Dental Services.* HC(89)2

Department of Health (2001a) *The Essence of Care: Patient focused benchmarking for health care.* DoH, London

Department of Health (2001b) *Extended prescribing of prescription only medicines by independent nurse prescribers* (MLX 273). Policy Unit — Executive Support, London

Department of Health (2001c) *Free toothpaste and toothbrushes for one million children.* Press release. DoH, London

Downer MC (1998) The changing pattern of dental disease over 50 years. *Br Dent J* **185**: 36–41

Durward C, Thou T (1997) Dental caries and sugar-containing liquid medicines for children in New Zealand. *N Z Dent J* **93**(414): 124–9

Eldridge K, Gallagher JE (2000) Dental caries prevalence and dental health behaviours in HIV infected children. *Int J Paed Dent* **10**: 19–26

Eyeson JD, Warnakulasuriya KAAS, Johnson NW (2000) Prevalence and incidence of oral lesions — the changing scene. *Oral Diseases* **6**(5): 267–73

Fiske J, Davis DM, Frances C, Gelbier S (1998) The emotional effects of tooth loss in edentulous people. *Br Dent J* **184**: 90–3

Fiske J, Griffeths J, Jamieson R, Manger D (2000) British Society for Disability and Oral Health guidelines for oral health care for long-stay patients and residents. *Gerontol* **17**(1): 55–64

Frank J, Drezner J (2001) Is teething in infants associated with fever or other symptoms? *J Family Pract* **50**(3): 257

Kelly M, Steele J *et al* (2000) *Adult Dental Health Survey: Oral Health in the United Kingdom, 1998.* The Stationery Office, London

Gallagher J (1998) Oral health needs: how can they be met? *Br J Community Nurs* **3**(1): 25–35

Greenspan D, Greenspan JS (1991) Management of oral lesions of HIV infection. *J Am Dent Assoc* **122**(9): 26–32

Health Education Authority (1996a) *A Handbook of Dental Health for Health Visitors, Midwives & Nurses.* 2nd edn. HEA, London

Health Education Authority (1996b) *The Scientific Basis of Dental Health Education.* 4th edn. HEA, London.

Health Education Authority (1998) *Birth to Five: The Health Education Authority's complete guide to the first five years of being a parent.* HEA, London

Hinds K, Gregory J (1995) *National diet and nutrition survey children aged 1 1/2 to 4 1/2 years Vol. 2 Report of the dental survey.* HMSO, London

Holt R, Murray JJ (1997) Developments in fluoride toothpastes — an overview. *Community Dent Health* **14**: 4–10

Hoppe JE (1997) Treatment of oropharyngeal candidosis in immunocompetent infants: a randomised multicenter study of miconazole gel vs nystatin suspension. The Antifungals Study Group. *Paediatr Infection Dis J* **16**(3): 288–93

Hulland SA, Lucas JO, Wake MA, Hesketh KD (2000) Eruption of the primary dentition in human infants: a prospective descriptive study. *Paediatric Dentistry* **22**(5): 415–21

Humphries JL, Green J (1999) *Nurse Prescribing*. Macmillan Press Ltd, Basingstoke

Johnson NW, ed (1991) *Risk Markers for Oral Diseases 2: Oral Cancer*. Cambridge University Press, Cambridge

Kay EJ, Locker D (1997) *Effectiveness of Oral Health Promotion: Health Promotion Effectiveness Review No 7*. Health Education Authority, London

Kelly M, Steele J, Nuttall *et al* (2000) *Adult Dental Health Survey, oral health in the United Kingdom, 1998*. TSO, London

Kent, Croucher R (1998) *Achieving Oral Health: The Social Context of Dental Care*. Wright, Oxford

King's Healthcare and LSLHA (1992) *Tooth tips for under fives: teething*. King's Healthcare, London

Locker D (1992) The burden of oral disorders in populations of older adults. *Community Dent Health* **9**(2): 109–24

Mackie IC, Bentley E (1994) Sugar-containing or sugar-free paediatric medicines: does it really matter? *Dent Update* **21**(5): 192–4

Macknin ML, Piedmonte M, Jacobs J, Skibinski C (2000) Symptoms associated with infant teething: a prospective study. *Paediatrics* **105**(4): 747–52

Maguire A, Rugg-Gunn AJ, Butler TJ (1996) Dental health of children taking antimicrobial and non-antimicrobial liquid oral medication long-term. *Caries Research* **30**(1):16–21

Munday P (1998) Strategies for community oral health promotion. *Br J Community Nurs* **3**(1): 36–40

National Prescribing Centre (1999) Signposts for prescribing nurses, general principles of good prescribing. *Prescrib Nurse Bull* **1**(1)

Nurse Prescribers' Formulary (1999) British Medical Association/Royal Pharmaceutical Society of Great Britain, London

Nuttall NM, Bradnock G, White D, Morris J, Nunn J (2001) Dental attendance in 1998 and implications for the future. *Br Dent J* **190**(4): 177–82

O'Brien M (1994) *Children's Dental Health in the United Kingdom, 1993*. HMSO, London

Paunovich ED, Aubertin MA, Saunders MJ, Prange M (2000) The role of dentistry in palliative care of the head and neck cancer patient. *Tex Dent J* **117**(6): 36–45

Pitts NB (1998) Inequalities in children's caries experience: the nature and size of the UK problem. *Community Dent Health* **15**(1): 296–300

Pitts NB, Evans DJ, Nugent (2001) The dental caries experience of 5-year-old children in the UK. Surveys co-ordinated by the British Association for the Study of Community Dentistry, 1999/2001. *Community Dent Health* **18**(1): 49–55

Pratelli P (2000) *Perceived Availability and Use of Dental Services by Adults with a Learning Disability Living in Private Households within Lambeth Southwark & Lewisham*. A report by the Department of Dental Public Health, King's College London for Lambeth, Southwark and Lewisham Health Authority. Unpublished

Royal Pharmaceutical Society of Great Britain (1997) *From Compliance to Concordance: Achieving Shared Goals in Medicine Taking*. RPS, London

Scully C, El-Kabir M, Samaranayake LP (1994) Candida and oral candidosis: a review. *Crit Rev Oral Biol Med* **5**(2): 125–57

Scully C, Cawson RA (1998) *Medical Problems in Dentistry*. 4th edn. Wright, Oxford

Secretary of State for Health (2000) *Modernising NHS Dentistry*. NHS Executive, London

Steele JG, Sheiham A, Marcenes W, Walls AWG (1998) *National Diet and Nutrition Survey; adults aged 65 and over*. HMSO, London

Steele J, Treasure E, Pitts NB, Morris J, Bradnock G (2000) Total tooth loss in the United Kingdom in 1998 and implications for the future. *Br Dent J* **189**(11): 598–603

Steward M (1988) Infant care: teething troubles. *Community Outlook* May: 27–8

Sweeney MP, Bagg (2000) The mouth and palliative care. *Am J Hosp Palliat Care* **17**(2): 118–24

Sweeney PC, Nugent Z, Pitts NB (1999) Deprivation and dental caries status of 5-year-old children in Scotland. *Community Dent Oral Epidemiol* **27**(2): 152–9

Sprod A, Anderson R, Treasure ET (1996) *Effective Oral Health Promotion: Literature Review.* Technical Report No 20. Health Promotion, Cardiff

Tiller S, Wilson KI, Gallagher JE (2001) Oral health status and dental service use of adults with learning disabilities living in residential institutions and in the community. *Community Dent Health* **18**(3): 167–71

Wake M, Hesketh K, Lucas J (2000) Teething and tooth eruption in infants: a cohort study. *Paediatrics* **106**(6): 1374–9

Warnakulasuriya KAAS, Johnson NW, Linklater KM, Bell J (1999) Cancer of mouth, pharynx and nasopharynx in Asian and Chinese immigrants resident in Thames regions. *Oral Oncol* **35**: 471–5

World Health Organization (1993) EC-Clearing house on Oral Problems related to HIV infection. WHO collaborating centre on Oral Manifestations of the immunodeficiency virus 22: 289–91

13

Informal peer support: a key to success for nurse prescribers

Christine Otway

A study was conducted in Leicestershire and Rutland (NHS) Healthcare Trust to determine the continuing professional development needs of nurse prescribers. Qualitative and quantitative approaches were applied to the sample frame of 350 nurse prescribers to elicit the most significant factors which have influenced the development of nurse prescribing. The majority of nurse prescribers considered prescribing to be a skill, which is now an essential part of core practice. The study indicated that informal peer support seems to have compensated for the absence of formal clinical supervision. Any development such as nurse prescribing has the added benefit of examining practice from new perspectives. Reflection on how this was achieved highlights important issues as to how the next stage can be even more successful.

The Medicinal Products: Prescription by Nurses etc Act 1992 allowed district nurses (DNs), health visitors (HVs) and practice nurses (PNs) who held either the DN or HV qualification, to prescribe from a limited formulary. Following successful evaluation of the pilot sites (Luker *et al*, 1997), the government allocated funds for the training of all eligible nurses in order to proceed towards full implementation of nurse prescribing. In May 2000, as the debate continued around the further extension of nurse prescribing, NHS Executive (NHS E) Trent had the foresight to fund a study to determine the continuing professional development (CPD) needs of nurse prescribers.

Leicestershire and Rutland (NHS) Healthcare Trust (LRHT) was the Trent regional pilot site for the implementation of nurse prescribing. This study was undertaken in this area because the trust had the benefit of employing nurses who had been qualified prescribers for over three years at the start of the data collection period. This was advantageous because experienced as well as less experienced nurse prescribers were able to recount the ways in which they had been supported during their training and after qualifying as prescribers. The benefit of experience enabled the nurses to reflect on their early development as prescribers and this provided qualitative data, which were used to determine CPD needs.

One of the most positive findings from the study was that the majority of nurse prescribers were confident and competent. The most significant support system for them was informal peer support and this had compensated for the lack of some of the more formalised structures of providing CPD, such as clinical supervision or mentorship. This chapter examines these issues in detail and then applies this knowledge to anticipate how support mechanisms might be improved both for existing and future independent and supplementary prescribers.

Background

I am a nurse prescriber, and qualified in the first cohort of nurse prescribers at De Montfort University in 1997. Since that time I have been employed by LRHT as an HV community practice teacher (CPT) and nurse prescriber and was seconded to De Montfort University for a year to undertake this study. My practical experience as a nurse prescriber meant that I had personal knowledge of the area I was researching. My own attitudes and perceptions were inevitably brought into the study, as are those of any researcher working within his/her own field. This can be an advantage because the issues are more easily understood, but can also mean that some of the more routine issues could be overlooked because of over-familiarity with them (Strauss and Corbin, 1990). It was also possible that the study may be biased because I was too close to the subject area (Robson, 1998). These facts were considered before and during data collection and to avoid overt bias I enlisted the help of other researchers, who were not prescribers, to aid in the study design and data analysis. The study was guided and supported by a steering group made up of representatives from key stakeholders in the implementation and development of nurse prescribing at both local and national level — the English National Board, the National Prescribing Centre, and local NHS Executive, NHS trusts and universities.

Design

The study used a survey design, organised in two phases. Phase 1 involved an in-depth investigation incorporating semi-structured interviews (*Box 13.1*) with twelve nurse prescribers.

Box 13.1. Semi-structured interview questions

- ❖ How long have you been a nurse prescriber?
- ❖ How useful is nurse prescribing to you as a professional, and to your clients?
- ❖ How often do you prescribe?
- ❖ Do you prescribe a variety of items from the *NPF* or just a few?
- ❖ What are these and why in your particular role are they useful?
- ❖ Should the *NPF* be extended?
- ❖ How do you keep yourself updated with changes to the *NPF*?
- ❖ Do you see pharmaceutical representatives (reps)?
- ❖ How useful are reps?
- ❖ Are you able to critically appraise the information they give you?
- ❖ Do you have regular clinical supervision?
- ❖ If yes, does it cover nurse prescribing issues?
- ❖ Could you give me an example of how it has helped your practice develop?
- ❖ What do you need to help you to develop your nurse prescribing skills?
- ❖ Who or what resources could help you with this? How? Why?
- ❖ How well do you know your local pharmacist or pharmacy adviser?
- ❖ How often do you use his/her expertise? Or how often would you if you could?
- ❖ Do you feel confident that you prescribe in a cost efficient way?
- ❖ Does this matter to you?
- ❖ Does your area have or is it developing a wound care formulary?

NPF = Nurse Prescribers' Formulary

These twelve were selected in order to provide an even geographical spread across the trust. Six were selected who were identified as active prescribers and six were identified as less active. Categories of active and less active were derived from database information about length of time qualified as prescribers and date of ordering their last prescription pad. The twelve nurse prescribers were provided with the opportunity to describe their own experiences of prescribing, the difficulties they faced, and any barriers which prevented them from prescribing effectively. Participants were assured of confidentiality at each stage of the process. These data were then analysed using thematic content analysis (Burnard, 1991) and the results were used to formulate phase 2.

Phase 2 consisted of self-completed questionnaires mailed to all 350 nurse prescribers employed by the trust, with a response rate of 69%. Questionnaires requested mainly quantitative data although some questions provided room for text replies and some respondents added text replies to supplement their answers. The forty questions were around the themes shown in *Box 13.2*.

The combined data from the two phases provided a wide and rich account of the experiences and difficulties faced by nurse prescribers and the analysis of this information gave a quantitative picture of their prescribing practice and indicated their CPD needs.

Box 13.2: Themes of phase 2 questionnaire

❖ Job title
❖ Length of time since qualifying
❖ Perceptions of usefulness of prescribing both to nurses and to patients
❖ Frequency of prescribing
❖ Isolation *vs* team working
❖ Confidence
❖ Support systems
❖ PREP requirements
❖ Cost and clinical effectiveness
❖ Information systems
❖ CPD needs

Results

Frequency and benefits of prescribing

Phase 1 showed that the most enthusiastic and active nurse prescribers were DNs. They tended to prescribe between six and ten times each day.

> *Essential, for dressings because working here my GPs are elsewhere in the town so to have to run after them for prescriptions would be an absolute nightmare.*

> (DN1)

HVs and PNs who tended to prescribe on average once or twice a week were also positive about the benefits of prescribing:

> *I can… immediately treat minor conditions. Also I can treat underlying skin dryness, which is preventative.*

(HV1)

This HV found that prescribing had definitely enhanced her practice:

> *We run a minor ailment session every day from 8.30 am till 11.00 am. We see babies and children with minor things. They are either self-referred or referred… by the doctor. We have this session every day so the clients know they can come to us for things and we tend to prescribe a lot.*

(HV2)

Teamwork and peer support

Analysis of the phase 1 qualitative data showed that more active prescribers tended to work in teams which included other nurse prescribers. These teams were described as cohesive and supportive. There were adequate opportunities for peer group support and sharing of information and experiences, which team members did not regard as formal support:

> *A lot of informal support and we certainly talk through incidents… we don't do [reflective practice] formally… but we do it. I think we miss out when we are short-staffed.*

(DN1)

This comment indicated that the informality of peer support meant that it happened anyway and that formal structures such as clinical support were not happening when workload increased or teams were short of staff.

Less active prescribers described themselves as being isolated from their peers:

> *I suppose I'd really like more interaction with other nurse prescribers, I haven't had any since I qualified as a nurse prescriber.*

(PN1)

There was clearly a wish to improve the situation from some practice nurses.

> *There are four of us here, but there are practice nurses...*
> *who work alone and are quite isolated... [at] the last PCG*
> *meeting, they are talking about actually closing down*
> *practices for half a day occasionally so people can... meet*
> *up with other nurses and other disciplines... there is quite*
> *a lot of isolation so there may be an opportunity in the*
> *future to change that.*

(PN2)

Isolation in practice seemed to be a significant negative factor, which had not been overcome by any formal support structures. Nurse prescribers who said that they lacked confidence in prescribing had often worked in isolated practices when they qualified as a nurse prescriber and they had not had time to consolidate their prescribing skills. This HV seemed very anxious about prescribing:

> *It's probably down to a lack of confidence on my part but*
> *when I do write prescriptions, because I don't do many I*
> *do worry a bit at the time. I need to get it right, I've got a*
> *checklist and I go over it and over it.*

(HV3)

Clinical supervision

Only two out of the twelve nurse prescribers interviewed in phase 1 were having regular formal clinical supervision. Although most of the nurses interviewed were aware of and understood the benefits of clinical supervision, it seemed that it was viewed as a luxury one could only afford when one was in a fully staffed and less pressured working situation:

> *We have team meetings, which we did use for clinical*
> *supervision but... its gone a bit by the board.*

(DN3)

Formal clinical supervision had not been implemented in the LRHT in 1997 when nurse prescribing was rolled out in the trust. The short timescale when the trust became a pilot site for nurse prescribing meant that the framework of clinical supervision, which was recommended in the implementation advice (NHS E, 1998) was not available in many areas. Some pilot sites, eg. West Midlands, set up clinical supervision specifically for their staff, using pharmacists as supervisors, in order to support nurse prescribing (Blenkinsopp and Savage, 1999).

At the time the study took place, LRHT was in the process of implementing clinical supervision using a 'bottom up' approach. There were no special arrangements, however, for clinical supervision to specifically support nurse prescribing. It was thought that clinical supervision would develop and would naturally incorporate issues involving prescribing as a part of core practice.

The study indicated that although many nurse prescribers believed that clinical supervision could help improve their prescribing practice, they had not been able to access it because their locations were short-staffed.

We do reflective practice but not clinical supervision.

(DN4)

One active nurse prescriber had regular reflective practice sessions with her peer group. She kept a duplicate book to record all her prescriptions, so was then able to reflect on her practice and double-check on prescriptions. One less active nurse prescriber said she reflected alone on her practice but was hoping that she could soon have clinical supervision as she felt that this would help her practice. Another respondent used to have reflective practice sessions but had to abandon them because her base was short-staffed. She now reflects alone but commented:

... clinical supervision [is] much better with someone else. It isn't always about finding answers.

(DN3)

A PN also indicated how clinical supervision would help her:

As I am working on my own its easy not to question yourself so clinical supervision would be useful... its good to have support... The GPs just think it's OK to let us get on with it but it would be nice to just talk to others about it from time to time.

(PN3)

Results from phase 2 of the study showed that, at the time the data collection took place, 52% of nurse prescribers were having clinical supervision regularly. Those who were receiving clinical supervision were asked whether these sessions covered prescribing issues: 48% answered 'yes'. Respondents were also asked about whether they thought group clinical supervision would help their prescribing practice, to which exactly half answered 'yes'. Several respondents added text to indicate that they planned to start clinical supervision soon in their area or to say that their sessions could cover prescribing issues but had not yet done so.

Mentorship

The plan in LRHT was that CPTs would be trained as nurse prescribers in the first cohort and would then be able to mentor future cohorts of nurse prescribers.

A mentor shares their student's experience, teaches the best way of doing things, enhances their protégée's skills and furthers their intellectual ability.

(Butterworth and Faugier, 1997)

Although CPTs possessed skills of mentorship they were not expert prescribers in the initial stages of the project because they had only been prescribing for a few weeks when the second and third cohorts trained. It could be argued therefore that they were not sufficiently skilled themselves to be able to teach adequately someone else the best way of doing something. Although mentorship skills are transferable (ENB, 2001), mentors need to develop and demonstrate sound professional knowledge and skills in that area before accepting responsibility as a mentor.

Luker *et al* (1997) recommended that in advance of the national roll-out of nurse prescribing, an advance-training programme be arranged at regional level for a few nurses from each area who could be used locally as mentors for nurse prescribing. It was envisaged that these nurses could provide support and input to the taught component of the nurse prescribing course and the study groups. This recommendation was not implemented and I could find no evidence to explain why not. It could be argued that this omission had had a significant impact on those nurse prescribers who had found difficulty in developing their prescribing skills, but for the majority it had not been significant.

The majority (95%) of respondents in phase 2 indicated that they had not had a mentor when they first started prescribing. The mentor is clearly a key factor in the provision of the learning environment. Adult learning has been described as transforming experience into knowledge, skills and attitudes (Jarvis, 1987). Kolb (1984) also described learning as a process whereby knowledge is created by the transformation of experience. The role of the mentor in this process is therefore to aid the transformation of experience into knowledge; it can be seen that in the absence of a mentor or any opportunity to reflect on experience, one may well be denied an important part of the process of learning. If these theories are correct one might assume that the introduction of nurse prescribing had been a disastrous failure. The study demonstrated, however, that this is certainly not the case for the majority of prescribers, who described themselves as being either confident or very confident in practice.

Educational evaluation

All learning stems from experience (Jarvis, 1997) and it is therefore difficult to assess the effectiveness of a practical skill such as nurse prescribing using a theoretical form of assessment. At the time that nurse prescribers were examined and deemed fit to practice they had never actually written a prescription. There had been no practical experience of prescribing in the course curriculum which might have aided their learning experience. As the initial evaluation looked only at pass rates it did not measure success in terms of its application to practice. Today's new prescribers have experienced prescribers to contact for advice, yet competency assessment for prescribing is still based on an examination.

Conclusion

This study has demonstrated that the informal peer group has been the significant support system, which has formed an essential part of the process of learning.

A peer is a colleague who is of similar status within the organization; someone who forms a collaborative relationship that is often mutually rewarding and non-competitive in nature.

(Morton-Cooper and Palmer, 1993)

The peer group in the study was made up of nurse prescribers with varying lengths and qualities of experience, including the initial cohort of CPTs. It could be argued that a significant majority of the sample would have been reflective practitioners, since reflective practice has been part of PREP requirements since 1995 (UKCC, 1995) and training has incorporated reflective practice for the past decade. The study shows that their informal capacity to reflect in and on action (Schon, 1983) and share experiences in an informal way with their peers appears to have been central to the way in which nurse prescribing has successfully developed. A limitation of this study was that it did not demonstrate the extent to which nurse prescribers considered themselves to be reflective practitioners.

Another recent study, which looked at support systems for nurse prescribers who were newly qualified, identified that peer support was thought by nurse prescribers to be a significant element of support (Humphries and Green, 2000). Earlier evaluations of nurse prescribing (Luker *et al*, 1997; Blenkinsopp *et al*, 1998) recognised the importance of clinical supervision and mentorship but did not acknowledge the significance of informal peer support.

This study had the benefit of focusing its research activity around a group of experienced nurse prescribers. The evidence shows that even when clinical supervision is implemented it is often the first thing to be cancelled when other pressures escalate. Informal peer support, however, is frequently still available even in times of stress and increased workloads. Cohesive and supportive teams are a valuable asset to the development of innovative practice. Unfortunately, constructive and supportive informal peer support is not available to every nurse.

Recommendations

Nurse prescribing presented nurses with a significant change to their core practice, which most welcomed and developed enthusiastically. However, health care is becoming more complicated and change more rapid, making more exacting demands on nurses. In some respects all nurses are agents of change and many of them acquire the skills needed intuitively (Kershaw, 1990). Others need more support in a planned and constructive environment.

In order to develop prescribing practice safely and effectively in the future it is important that responsibility for its development takes place at an organisational level. It is suggested that nurse prescribers will need to have skilled mentors and good informal peer support systems as well as regular clinical supervision. In order to ensure that these systems are actually in place it is suggested that a group, known as a prescribing support forum, is specifically charged with this responsibility. Prescribing support forums would be formed in each primary care trust. It is suggested that forums are made up of:

- an experienced nurse prescriber
- a GP
- a pharmacist.

This group needs to be aware of nurses who are prescribing in isolation in order to ensure that formalised support structures are in place that support and develop their prescribing practice.

The prescribing support forum also needs to have clear and reliable links with local academic institutions so that the nurse prescribers of the future are given the best theoretical and practical education and CPD to prepare them for and support them during their professional working lives.

Although this study has looked specifically at nurse prescribing, the lessons learned can be applied to many other areas where nurses are extending their scope of practice (UKCC, 1992). More attention needs to be paid to the teams that exist in healthcare settings and work needs to be done to ensure that their informal success is translated into formal support for professional practice.

Key Points

- ⌘ Nurse prescribers in this study had been qualified for up to three years.
- ⌘ Prescribing had been successful despite variable provision of support systems.
- ⌘ Isolated working needs to be overcome by formal support systems.

References

Blenkinsopp A, Grime J, Pollock K, Boardman H (1998) *Nurse Prescribing Evaluation 1: The Initial Training Programme and Implementation*. Department of Medicines Management, Keele University

Blenkinsopp A, Savage I (1999) *Nurse Prescribing Evaluation 2: Continuing Development Needs*. Department of Medicines Management, Keele University

Burnard P (1991) A method of analysing interview transcripts in qualitative research. *Nurse Educ Today* **11**: 461–6

Butterworth T, Faugier J (1997) *Clinical Supervision and Mentorship in Nursing*. Chapman & Hall, London

English National Board for Nursing, Midwifery and Health Visiting (2001) *Preparation of Mentors and Teachers: A New Framework of Guidance*. ENB, London

Humphries J, Green E (2000) Nurse prescribers: infrastructures required to support their role. *Nurs Standard* **14**(48): 35–9

Jarvis P (1997) *Adult Learning in the Social Context*. Croom Helm, London

Kolb D (1984) *Experiential Learning: Experience as a Source of Learning and Development*. Prentice-Hall, Englewood Cliffs (NJ)/London

Kershaw B (1990) *Nursing Competence: A Guide to Professional Development*. Edward Arnold, London, Melbourne, Auckland

Luker K, Austin L, Hogg C, Ferguson B, Smith K (1997) *Evaluation of Nurse Prescribing: Final Report*. The University of Liverpool and the University of York

Morton-Cooper A, Palmer A (1993) *Mentoring and Preceptorship: A Guide to Support Roles in Clinical Practice*. Blackwell Scientific Publications, Oxford

National Health Service Executive (1998) *Nurse Prescribing: A Guide for Implementation*. NHS E, Leeds

Robson C (1998) *Real World Research*. Blackwell, Oxford

Schon D (1983) *The Reflective Practitioner: How Professionals Think in Action*. Basic Books, New York

Strauss A, Corbin J (1990) *Basics of Qualitative Research*. Sage Publications, London

United Kingdom Central Council for Nursing, Midwifery and Health Visiting (1992) *The Scope of Professional Practice*. UKCC, London

United Kingdom Central Council for Nursing, Midwifery and Health Visiting (1995) *Standards for Post-registration Education and Practice*. UKCC, London

14

Caring for dry and damaged skin in the community

Jill Peters

Community nurses are ideally place to fully utilise nurse prescribing to improve the accessibility to emollient therapy for any patient with dry skin, regardless of cause. Skin diseases affect 23% of the general population and patients accessing care in the primary setting contribute to 15–20% of general practice appointments.

The current nurse prescribing course is an introduction to prescribing but the actual decision making of diagnosis and choice of therapy is based on clinical knowledge, cost effectiveness, and experience of previous use and is part of the ongoing professional development that every nurse prescriber undertakes.

It is hoped that this chapter will facilitate greater understanding of the therapeutic effect of dermatological products for dry and damaged skin so that prescribing nurses can make appropriate choices, and patients' access to the treatment they require and clinical and quality of life outcomes can be improved. Unfortunately, there is little evidence to enable recommendation of one product over another and several factors have to be considered when making the choice of product. The best emollient is the one the patient likes and uses.

To understand the care needed for dry and damaged skin we need to consider the function of the skin to identify why skin becomes dry and damaged.

Anatomy and physiology

The skin comprises three layers: the epidermis (outer layer); dermis (corium layer); and subcutaneous tissue (subcutis) (*Figure 14.1*). It is a continuous sheath that covers the outside of the body and weighs one-sixth of total body weight.

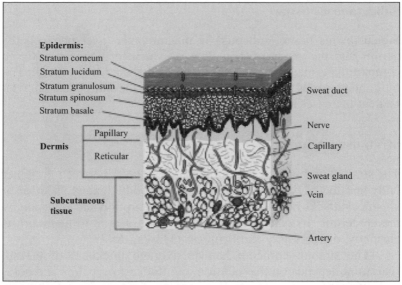

Figure 14.1: Cross-section of the skin showing major structures and layers

Epidermis

As *Figure 14.1* shows, the epidermis contains no blood vessels of its own but takes its nutrition from the dermis. The intercellular space of the epidermis is filled with lymph so when injured it does not bleed but oozes. Adjacent cells are attached to each other by desomosomes as flexible adhesive junctions. The desomosomes stabilise the epidermis and attach to the dermis.

Dermis

The dermis (corium) is composed of collagenous and elastic fibres. This makes the dermis very elastic and is responsible for its great tensile strength. It is distensible and can contract. The water binding capacities of the collagenous fibres and ground substance (consisting of polysaccharides and protein (Ebling *et al*, 1992) are responsible for the tonicity of the skin.

Subcutaneous tissue

Subcutaneous tissue (subcutis) is the movable layer between the dermis and the general fascia. It is a system of connective tissue compartments made of collagenous fibres that are filled with fat. The fat content varies based on the location on the body. A higher fat content increases skin tension.

Stratum corneum

The stratum corneum is the true protective layer between the inner body and the environment, defending the body against physical or chemical attacks but also limiting water absorption and emission by the epidermis. Its water binding ability is essential to maintain its elasticity, distensibility and firmness (Marks, 1997).

The stratum corneum has an average thickness of 0.1mm (variation depends on the location, eg. thickest on palms and soles and thinnest on the face). It consists of approximately twenty compacted layers of flattened horny cells called keratinocytes. The keratinocytes derive from cells formed by cell division at the stratum basale which gradually migrate to the surface, undergoing change at every level until they reach the stratum corneum and die. The upper layers of keratinocytes are sloughed off continually in a process called desquamation.

From cell division in the stratum basale to desquamation takes twenty-eight days, of which fourteen are required for the process of keratinization. This involves the transformation of living keratinocytes into dead horny material; the water content and protein of the cells is reabsorbed and the cytoplasm is replaced by the insoluble protein keratin.

Keratin is not the only substance found in the stratum corneum; it also has non-keratin by-products from the keratinization process. These substances can bind and retain water in the stratum corneum and are known as natural moisturising factors (NMFs) (Cork, 1997), the most important of which are lactic acid, pyrrolidonecarboxylic acid, urea, urocannic acid and carbohydrates bound to scleroproteins. Perspiration is another mechanism by which the stratum corneum is moistened.

If the NMFs are removed from the stratum corneum it looses its capacity to bind water. Known causes for removal of NMFs from the epidermis:

- extensive washing of skin with soap — accumulative
- soap not washed off the skin surface
- extensive soaking in water — over twenty minutes immersed.

Deeper within the stratum corneum, the cells are held together securely but elastically by a fat-like cement substance called glycoprotein intercellular substance (Savin *et al*, 1989).

The hydrolipid film

The surface of the stratum corneum is covered by a continually renewed hydrolipid film, composed of a mixture of water and fats (Alonso *et al*, 1996). The hydrolipid film consists of:

- lipids from sebaceous gland secretion (sebum)
- water (perspiration)
- proteins
- salts from sweat glands.

Three stratum corneum lipids — ceramides, cholesterol and free fatty acids — are required for permeable barrier homeostasis (Mao-Qiang *et al*, 1996).

This natural emulsion depends on the levels of lipid and water within. It is either an oil in water (o/w) or a water in oil (w/o) emulsion. The amount of hydrolipid film produced by the skin is determined genetically but is also subject to circadian rhythms and depends on the time of year (eg. increases in higher temperatures) as well as the climate (Cork, 1997; Van de Kerkhof, 1997).

Hormones also play a role in regulating hydrolipid film production. Androgen hormones stimulate while estrogen, progesterone and the corticosteroids inhibit production of the hydrolipid film.

Age also influences the production levels of the hydrolipid film. It is low before puberty, then increases sharply during puberty and decreases after the age of thirty-five. The emulsion changes most dramatically in old age. The reduction in sweat and sebaceous gland secretion as well as water loss through the skin results in true deficiency that the body can no longer compensate for. The skin dries out and becomes sensitive to chemicals, eg. alkaline soaps (Cork, 1997; Van de Kerkhof, 1997).

The hydrolipid film, together with the water barrier of the lower stratum corneum, is crucial to the condition of the skin. The natural emulsion keeps the epidermis smooth and supple. On the outside it is a water repellent and hinders the penetration of water-soluble substances and on the inside it protects the skin from drying out.

The hydrolipid film also produces a protective acid coating on the skin. It is usually a slightly acidic pH 4.5–5.75 (Hughes, 2001). This gives the skin a protective coating against the affects of alkaline solution and indirectly against attacks from bacteria and fungi. Excessive washing can destroy this protective coating.

Circadian rhythms

There has been little work so far on Circadian rhythms and the physiopathology of the skin but patients often mention feeling hot and itchier in the evenings. New studies (Yosipovitch *et al*, 1998) demonstrated marked circadian differences noted in skin temperature, transepidermal water loss (TEWL) and skin surface pH. Of these changes, TEWL may have the greatest impact pharmacologically when you consider the epidermal barrier decreases during this time, and thus the topical drug permeability may increase significantly (Yosipovitch *et al*, 1998). Future work could look at the recommendation of an emollient and therapeutic preparations should be applied to the skin in the evening to ensure maximum benefit by absorption. As the skin temperature also increases this would explain the exacerbation of pruritus in the late afternoon and evening.

Young skin

Dry skin in babies and toddlers occurs because the skin as an organ is not fully developed although all the structures are in place. The newborn dermis is less mature, with less organised vascular and nerve structures, collagen and elastic fibres than an adult. The dermis does not form like an adult's until the age of two years (Weston and Lane, 1991).

In children under two years old, the whole skin is one-fifth thinner and the stratum corneum is thinner and weaker than adult skin. The keratin cells are not so tightly packed so the skin's protective function is less. It also means that greater absorption of topical medication can occur as children also have a greater relative body surface area (Atherton, 1994; Greaves and Gatti, 1999).

This immaturity means that the hydrolipid film and protective acid coating is not fully developed (the sebaceous glands are not fully developed until puberty). Children's skin therefore has less capability to protect itself from drying and alkaline substances.

The adolescent's skin undergoes dramatic change when puberty commences as a result of an increase of hormone production. Adolescents also undergo psychological changes such as increased awareness of sexual attraction and become concerned with how others perceive them. They often rebel against taking responsibility for emollient therapy. This should not necessarily be interpreted simply as non-compliance but as a response to self-discovery (Turnbull, 2001).

Older skin

The skin in older people is more likely to be dry because of the physiological changes that occur with aging — sweat and sebum secretion decrease and the hydrolipid film is not so protective. Over the age of sixty the epidermis thins by 50% and there is a loss of elasticity and turgor of the skin as the dermis loses its normal fibrous structure and the collagenous fibres lose the ability to bind water (Van de Kerkhof, 1997).

External factors also play a major role in damaging older skin. Accumulation of sun exposure damages the skin's DNA so that it can no longer repair itself (Van de Kerkhof, 1997). Excessive exposure to soap and frequency of washing over time deplete the hydrolipid film and it is unable to replenish itself sufficiently to maintain a protective barrier (Van de Kerkhof, 1997). Combined with the dry atmosphere created by central heating this depletion often leads to dry, cracked skin.

Damaged skin

Damage to skin frequently occurs when detergents or organic solvents remove lipids from the surface of the skin. The skin loses its ability to compensate through its own lipid formation mechanism. Too much cleansing of the skin removes not only lipids from the surface but also washes away the NMFs.

This process makes the skin rough and dry. Dry skin tends to scale and becomes itchy. Further damage is done by the scratching; scratching stimulates the release of proinflammatory mediators such as histamine, which makes itching worse and potentially leading to the development of eczematous lesions (Cork, 1997). These in turn increase the risk of infection. When infected the local area becomes flooded with serous fluid and moisture causing the stratum corneum to swell and so increasing its sensitivity. If there is extensive oedema then blistering can occur as in cellulitis.

Healthy skin can take on the characteristics of eczematous skin when experimentally damaged in the laboratory using a 'scratching machine' (Bridgett *et al*, 1996). Lichenified (thickened) skin can be also seen where two skin surfaces have rubbed against one another.

Patients with venous insufficiency will have low-lipid skin (Williams, 1996). As compression bandages prevent shedding of the stratum corneum these patients will often have visible keratinocytes on the surface of the skin. The skin appears very dry and when the bandages or support stocking are removed, skin can flake off or remain on the skin surface and require moisturising before it can be picked off.

Inflammatory dermatoses

Alterations in the epidermal lipids in atopic eczema result in a defective epidermal barrier and loss of water from the stratum . As a result, the corneocytes shrink and cracks open between them that permit passage of irritants or allergens (Cork, 1997).

Dry skin is also caused by inflammatory processes within the skin resulting from a range of causes (dermatoses, infections, trauma, chemical burns) or due to disturbances during the keratinization process (psoriasis) (*Box 14.1*).

> **Box 14.1: Conditions causing dry skin**
>
> ❖ Atopic eczema
> ❖ Psoriasis
> ❖ Contact dermatitis
> ❖ Varicose eczema
> ❖ Eczema craqulé

Topical emollient therapy has been found to make a significant difference to the management dermatoses. Use of emollients in eczema reduces itching, improves the condition of the skin and may avoid the use of topical steroids (Rajka, 1997). Here the health visitor can give advice to parents of children who have dry skin to improve the hydrolipid barrier, reducing the possibility of antigens passing through and triggering the atopic cycle. The district nurse who proactively promotes emollient therapy with the over-sixties may also help reduce the dryness and itchiness that can be so distressing.

Emollient therapy can also improve the condition of psoriasis as it can both soothe the skin so it is more flexible and reduce discomfort and fissuring. More importantly for the patient, emollient therapy can improve psoriasis cosmetically by reducing scaling (Finlay, 1997).

Skin assessment

Before effective emollient therapy can be started, a full examination should be carried out. Examination should be conducted in a warm, private room with good natural or artificial lighting that will not change the natural colour of the skin (Lawton, 1998). A good magnifying lamp is useful when assessing lesions; this allows the use of perpendicular lighting when looking for subtle skin changes. In the patient's home, use natural lighting where possible otherwise take a small portable light with a magnifying lens with you.

The assessment — which must take into account psychological as well as physical aspects of the patient's condition — should start at the onset of patient/nurse meeting: consider the patient's physical bearing and posture. Slouching posture, avoidance of eye contact or shyness could indicate unhappiness, loss of self-esteem or self-confidence, anger or embarrassment (Bates, 1995). Their expectations of treatment may be high and care must be taken to explain why they have a skin problem, and what realistic aims of treatment are — in dermatology terms we discuss remission and control but rarely cure.

An unhappy child who is distressed, irritated and appears unwell is a good indicator of the systemic effects of the inflammatory disease process, eg. a child with acute atopic eczema is often visually distressed whereas a child with seborrhoea dermatitis is not (Turnbull, 1999).

Assessment of children is more complicated as you may have to communicate through parents/carers, but a structured assessment format is necessary to gain an accurate and detailed history (Turnbull, 2000). Allow the parents/carers to undress the child on their lap if necessary and ensure that your hands are warm. Warn the child that you are going to gently feel his/her skin. Check into all the skin folds, as parents often do not relate a rash on one part of the body to a rash on another part. Use the child health record to document and promote shared communication.

In all assessments, use of analogue scales (ie. 0–10 scales) can be a useful tool for documenting and re-evaluating skin conditions on review visits. Look at the epidermis; notice if individual skin cells are visible. Does the skin look scaly? How red (erythematous) is the skin, and to what degree, florid to pale pink? Touch the skin in several places. Is it hot to the touch? Does the skin feel dry or rough? Is there any change in pigmentation or lichenification? What is the turgor like? Are there any excoriations, fissures or epidermal changes, eg. inflammation? All these data need to be documented on a body chart to illustrate severity and distribution of the dry/damaged skin. This makes it easier to review the patient. It is also important to note down any improvements the patient comments on such as, 'I am less itchy' or, 'I am sleeping better'.

Prescribing emollients

When prescribing an emollient therapy the following should be considered:

- patient preference of greasiness on the skin
- severity of dryness of their skin
- known sensitivities
- patient's dexterity
- carer's preference
- mobility
- safety in the bathroom (rubber mats in the bath or shower)
- cost-effectiveness.

Choice

Although empirical research demonstrates the effectiveness of emollient therapy through measurement of water loss (TEWL), electrical parameters and visual analogue scales (Marks, 1997) comparison studies between actual products are extremely rare. Studies are usually done comparing an emollient product with cosmetic products (Hardy, 1996), eg. E45 and two liquid soaps as cited by Marks (1997). This should be an area for further research to demonstrate what is the best emollient for each situation. Unfortunately, each human being is unique and therefore what is effective and suitable for one patient may not be for another.

Choice, therefore, may be based on previous usage by patient as well as the eight points listed above. There is a range of products available. It is advisable to have samples of each emollient available at the clinic or base; this means the patient can try each product there and then. It is then possible to negotiate with the patient their choice of product. This can avoid several different products being prescribed simultaneously and so reduce cost.

Emollient properties

Emollients available for prescription and over the counter come in several forms — creams, lotions, ointments, sprays, bath additives. Preparations may be light in texture with a high water content, or have a higher 'grease' content. Lighter preparations are absorbed quickly, and do not leave the skin feeling greasy, but they have a shorter period of effectiveness and so more frequent applications are needed (Marks, 1997). More greasy preparations will be more effective for very dry, fissured (cracked) skin because they have a lower quantity of water, and they have a longer effective period (Marks, 1997). However, patients may express concern over use of a greasier emollient because the greasiness can damage clothing and furniture. They feel embarrassed if they leave greasy marks where they have been.

Emollients provide an oily layer over the surface of the stratum corneum, which traps water underneath it. The water is held back and reabsorbed into the horny layer and as a result, reduces the fissuring (Cork, 1997). The emollient also mimics the barrier effect of the hydrolipid film when it penetrates into the upper layers of the stratum corneum (Cork, 1997). Emollients that contain all three stratum corneum lipids (ceramides, cholesterol and free fatty acids) promote barrier homeostasis following acute barrier disruption. Further acceleration can occur if any quantity of one of the three lipids is increased (Mao-Qiang *et al*, 1996).

All emollient products may have added ingredients either to keep them chemically stable (eg. preservatives) or to increase the specific action of the preparation (eg. urea). These added ingredients can act as allergens and provoke an immune response or sensitisation.

It is also important to be aware of potential side-effects: for example, stinging is common when using products that contain urea or lactic acid (Marks, 1997). Changing to a product without the component that caused the reaction/side-effect will make a difference. This is particularly important if trying to manage emollient therapy in children so that the experience is not unpleasant and more like fun and play to encourage concordance. The Monthly Index of Medical

Specialities (MIMS) has some very useful charts indicating what active ingredients are in different emollient products, which can assist in the decision about which product to prescribe.

It is important to explain to the patient what the role of the product is so that they understand why it is important to use it more than once a day.

Application

Explanation of application technique is essential to clinical improvement and comfort for the patient.

Bathing

Soap substitutes (eg. aqueous cream, emulsifying ointment, Epaderm) cleanse like soap but are non-drying and help hydrate the skin. Commercial pH-neutral cleansing products can also be used as they do not exacerbate dermatoses. They should be applied to the skin before getting into water, but make sure the hands are dry and not greasy and there is a rubber non-slip mat in the bath.

The water should be body temperature (tepid) (Hardy, 1996) to reduce dilation of blood vessels. Overly hot water causes excessive perspiration. It is useful to have a supply of soap substitute at every sink in the home.

Frequency of bathing can make a difference to the dryness of the skin, as well as length of time in the water (Hardy, 1996). Ideally a bath should be about ten minutes long, and definitely no longer than twenty minutes, otherwise the epidermis becomes waterlogged and the hydrolipid film is weakened, permeability increases and the skin becomes dryer. The skin should be patted dry not rubbed.

Bath oils (*Box 14.2*) should be used carefully, observing the recommended dose, as irritant reactions can occur if they contain an active agent, eg. an antiseptic (Ling and Highet, 2000). Excessive use of bath oils makes the bath very slippery.

Box 14.2: Some bath additives

❖ Alpha Keri Bath® (Bristol-Myers Squibb)
❖ Aveeno® (Bioglan Laboratories)
❖ Balneum® (Crookes Healthcare)
❖ Diprobath® (Schering-Plough)
❖ Emmolate® (Bio-Medical)
❖ Hydromol Emollient® (Quinoderm Ltd)
❖ Oilatum® preparations (Stiefel)

Applying to the skin

Topical emollients (*Box 14.3*) should be trialed by each patient, to find out how quickly their skin becomes dry and when should they reapply their emollient. Suggest that a moisturiser is applied hourly for three hours with the patient touching their skin at the end of each hour before reapplying the moisturiser. They should then be able to establish at what time lapse their skin became dry and use this as a guide to reapplication frequency throughout the day (Marks, 1997). Areas of exposed skin like face, neck and hands will dry out more quickly than covered areas, so more frequent applications will be required.

Box 14.3: Some topical emollients

❖ Alcoderm®(Galderm
❖ Dermamist® (spray) (Yamanouchi)
❖ Diprobase® (Schering-Plough)
❖ E45® (Crookes Healthcare)
❖ Epaderm® (Seton Scholl)
❖ Hydromol® (Quinoderm Ltd)

❖ Keri® (Bristol-Myers Squibb)
❖ LactiCare® (Stiefel)
❖ Neutrogena® Dermatological Cream (Johnson & Johnson)
❖ Oilatum® (Stiefel)
❖ Ultrabase® (Schering Health)
❖ Unguentum M® (Crookes Healthcare)

Often creams are preferred during the day as they are less greasy and do not leave a shine on the skin. Ointments can then be applied at night. Very few emollients are comedogenic (cause acne-like spots) because of the removal of cocoa butter derivatives from most products (Marks, 1997).

The applications should be light, a glisten on the skin, not a thick heavy application that damages the clothes or furniture. Apply in smooth downward strokes, in the direction of hair growth to reduce the possibility of poral occlusion and a form of miliaria (Marks, 1997). Gentle application should be used so as not to irritate the skin. Rubbing should be avoided, as it creates friction that could cause thickening of the epidermis.

Prescribing emollients

It is often useful to supply emollients in tubes or encourage the patients to decant the product from a large to a smaller container. The product can then be carried in bags or be in the drawer at work; easy access encourages concordance.

Products should not be shared if hands are dipping into a tub of cream. Tubs may contain skin scales and bacteria from the user, as bacteria will easily grow in a moist environment (Davis, 2001). Pump dispensers are cleaner and easy to use for patients with arthritis who cannot undo other containers.

When writing a prescription for an emollient, several other factors must be considered. Take care to prescribe sufficient quantities of the product: in cases of widespread generalised dryness, 50g a day can frequently be used.

Patient dexterity should also be considered. For those who have difficulty applying creams and ointments, a spray emollient is available. There are tools available that look like long-handled paint rollers with a washable plastic roller that can enable patients to moisturise their backs and lower legs.

If there has been no improvement of an older person's skin following emollient therapy then do consider metabolic deficiency that could be the cause of their dry itchy skin: low iron, thyroid dysfunction, liver disease are all possibilities, so a blood screen is essential.

Discuss with patients the environment in which they live because this may affect how dry their skin is. Central heating (Hardy, 1996), air conditioning (eg. inside of airplanes), and moving quickly between hot and cold environments all affect the skin. Extra emollient applications may be needed under these circumstances. During the hot summer months changing from a grease-based emollient to a water-based emollient may keep the skin cooler (Marks, 1997), and helps avoid sunburn if an emollient is applied before sun protection products.

Conclusion

Community nurses can offer patients access to the topical emollient therapy they need, in the quantities they require, by being proactive with prescribing. Through understanding the role of emollients in improving the condition of dry and damaged skin — and potentially the quality of life of the patient — the nurse has a key role in the education and support of these patients. Nurses themselves are at high risk of occupational dermatitis and should be proactive in the care of their own skin by using emollient therapy (Rycroft, 1997).

Key Points

- Concordance in emollient therapy is best achieved through explanation and negotiation.

- A good emollient is one that the patient prefers and uses.

- Only light applications are needed, so the skin glistens, with frequent reapplications.

References

Alonso A, Meirelles NC, Yushmanov VE, Tabak M (1996) Water increases the fluidity of intercellular membranes of stratum corneum: correlation with water permeability, elastic and electrical resistance properties. *J Invest Dermatol* **106**(5): 1058–63

Atherton DJ (1994) *Eczema in Childhood: the facts.* Oxford University Press, Oxford

Bates B (1995) *A Guide to Physical Examination and History Taking.* 6th edn. WW Lippincott, Philadelphia

Cork MJ (1997) The importance of skin barrier function. *J Dermatol Treatments* **8**(Suppl 1): 7–13

Davis R (2001) Treatment issues relating to dermatology. In: Hughes E, Van Onselen J, eds. *Dermatology Nursing A Practical Guide.* Churchill Livingstone, Edinburgh: 41–51

Ebling FJG, Eady RAJ, Leigh IM (1992) Anatomy and organization of human skin. In: Champion RH, Burton JL, Ebling FJG, eds. Rook/Wilkinson/Ebling *Textbook of Dermatology.* 5th edn. Blackwell, Oxford: 49–123

Finlay AY (1997) Emollients as adjuvant therapy for psoriasis. *J Dermatol Treatments* **8**(Suppl 1): 25–7

Greaves MW, Gatti S (1999) The use of glucocorticoids in dermatology. *J Dermatol Treatments* **10**: 83–91

Hardy MA (1996) What can you do about your patient's dry skin? *J Gerontol Nurs* **22**(5): 1018

Hughes (2001) Skin: its structure, function and related pathology. In Hughes E, Van Onselen J, eds. *Dermatology Nursing: A Practical Guide.* Churchill Livingstone, Edinburgh: 6

Lawton S (1998) Assessing the skin. *Prof Nurse* **13**(4 Suppl): S5–S7

Ling TC, Highet AS (2000) Irritant reactions to an antiseptic bath emollient. *J Dermatol Treatments* **11**: 263–7

Mao-Qiang M, Feingold KR, Thornfeldt CR, Elias PM (1996) Optimization of physiological lipid mixtures for barrier repair. *J Invest Dermatol* **106**(5): 1096–101

Marks R (1997) How to measure the effects of emollients. *J Treatments* **8**(Suppl 1): S15–S18

National Prescribing Centre (1999) Signposts for prescribing nurses: general principles of good prescribing. *Prescrib Nurse Bull* **1**(1): 1–4

Rajka G (1997) Emollient therapy in atopic dermatitis. *J Dermatol Treatments* **8**(Suppl 1): S19–S21

Rycroft RJG (1997) Occupational hand eczema: the role of emollients in treatment and prophylaxis. *J Dermatol Treatments* **8**(Suppl 1): S23–S24

Turnbull R (2000) Skin assessment in children: a methodical approach. *Nurs Times* **96**(41): 33–4

Turnbull R (2001) Puberty and the skin. *Br J Dermatol Nurs* **5**(2): 16–17

Van de Kerkhof PCM (1997) What are dry skin conditions? *J Dermatol Treatments* **8**(Suppl 1): S3–S5

Weston WL, Lane AT (1991) *Colour Textbook of Pediatric Dermatology*. Mosby, St. Louis

Williams (1996) Treatment of leg ulcers:1. *Br J Nurs* **5**(4): 208–15

Yosipovitch G, Xiong GL, Haus E, Sackett-Lundeen L, Ashkenazi I, Mailbach HI (1998) Time-dependent variations of the skin barrier function in humans: Transepidermal water loss, stratum corneum hydration, skin surface poH and skin temperature. *J Investigative Dermtatol* **110**(1): 20–3